the
ARTHRITIS
handbook

DARRELL C. CRAIN
M.D., F.A.C.P.

AN
ARC
BOOK

ARCO PUBLISHING COMPANY, INC.

219 Park Avenue South, New York, N.Y. 10003

An ARC Book
published 1972 by Arco Publishing Company, Inc.
219 Park Avenue South, New York, N.Y. 10003
by arrangement with Exposition Press, Inc.

Library of Congress Catalog Card Number 72-3319
ISBN 0-668-02685-5

Printed in the United States of America

Contents

PART THREE

Preface

The first edition of this book was published in 1959 under the title, *Help For Ten Million*. But that was apparently confusing, and many people—with characteristic impatience—never read the rest of the title, "A Manual for Patients With Arthritis, Rheumatism and Gout." So it seemed wise when making a revision to strike out boldly and tell at a glance what one might find between the covers. Hence, the new title.

Of more importance are the changes that have been made in the text. The entire chapter on Treatment (Chapter IX) has been rewritten. Not that any sure cure has been found—not yet. But the present method of presentation should assist the patient in organizing his attack on the disease. Changes, including the addition of diagrams, have been made in the appendix dealing with exercises. For them, I am indebted to Dr. Margaret Kenrick, director of the Department of Physical Medicine and Rehabilitation at Georgetown University School of Medicine. Also, a new chapter has been added on medical quackery.

To my sorrow, the death of Mr. Fred Kelly has denied me the editorial assistance in this edition which was of such great value in the first. Without his advice and encouragement, the book would never have been started, nor finished. I regret that he cannot share with me the pleasure and satisfaction of knowing that a second edition was needed, and has now been brought into existence.

Introduction

Today everyone is interested in arthritis. What a change from former years when it was the stepchild of scientific research. In 1938, when a group of farsighted doctors attempted to organize a national foundation for rheumatic diseases, there was so little interest among laymen *and doctors* that the plan had to be shelved. It seems difficult, now, to explain why true scientific research to determine causes and treatments for arthritis has been so slow to come. Probably one reason is that man is a selfish animal and seems more concerned about those diseases that are contagious. If several of our neighbors have an illness that we may catch, we insist that something be done about it. Rheumatism, not being communicable by association with others, was neglected. We felt sorry for those afflicted, but knew that their having it would not give it to us. So no effort was made to provide funds for the kind of research so badly needed.

Today, happily, that situation has changed. The Arthritis Foundation (which that same group of doctors who failed in 1938, finally got started ten years later) now raises millions of dollars annually, supports hundreds of clinics throughout the country, has granted dozens of research fellowships, and is carrying out an ever-expanding information program.

Our federal government, too, has taken up the torch. Whereas, in 1950, the Public Health Service was interested only in such problems as water purification, mosquito control and infectious diseases, its program now includes all phases of medicine. The great clinical center, in Bethesda, Maryland, a suburb of Washington, includes the National Institute of Arthritis and Metabolic Diseases which conducts investigations in clinical research and also administers grants to medical schools for research and teaching programs. All the large drug houses are conducting research to develop new and better medicines for treatment. And you—the millions of people to whom this book is addressed, the sufferers from arthritis and other rheumatic diseases—you have thus seen the dawn of an era when others have become interested in your problems and have resolved to give you help. This book, too, is intended to help you in your difficulties. It is not a "do-it-yourself" book—for the arthritic who tries to manage his own case will surely get into trouble. Rather, it is to be used as a manual under the direction of your physician—much as a student in a science class uses a manual with the help of the professor to solve a problem.

Each reader should find many things in this book that apply to his particular case. You will also, of course, find things that do not. Now, which things do, and which do not, can only be determined by a physician after a thorough study and complete evaluation of the individual problem. Then, after a diagnosis has been established, and your physician has found out what program your heart, lungs, liver and kidneys, can tolerate, he can advise you just what in this manual is for you.

It will be noted that the manual is divided into three parts. The first deals with the most important forms of true arthritis, and various miscellaneous rheumatic diseases; the second with gout. Although a person may be afflicted with more than one of these conditions at a time, nevertheless this division seems to be a practical one for most readers. Part three consists of three appendices dealing with diet, exercises, and mechanical aids.

One final word before getting on with the main issue: Remember that results are not always accomplished in a few days. Persons with arthritis must measure their treatment in weeks—or months. And it is at times necessary for the plan of treatment to be completely altered—for what helps one person may not help another, even if both have ills that seem identical. Your fight against arthritis can be likened to a struggle between two great armies. Where one has the upper hand, and is firmly entrenched, the tide of battle is turned with difficulty. But it can be done—just keep after it!

PART ONE

I It's an Old-Timer

Congratulations, arthritics, on your medical ancestry. Your disease is no Johnny-come-lately in the realm of medicine. On the contrary, it is a charter member of the Oldest Inhabitants Club. Long before Pandora's box was opened, her ancestors were complaining of painful joints. Even fossilized bones of dinosaurs, pterodactyls, and other vertebrate creatures that roamed the earth long before man arrived, show that they, too, were rheumatic. The ape man of the Pliocene age, millions of years ago, as well as the Neolithic man of a later period, suffered from stiffened joints. Studies of mummies show that the many predynastic Nubians and Egyptians must have had to go limping about from rheumatism. So did the earliest North American Indians. Luke, the physician, tells of ". . . a woman which had a spirit of infirmity eighteen years, and was bowed together, and could in no wise lift up herself" (Luke XIII. 11). Socrates, in Greece, listed arthritis first among the common diseases of his time. It was so prevalent in Rome that the Emperor Diocletian issued an edict exempting those most severely afflicted from the payment of taxes. Yes, your medical family tree goes back a long way.

Congratulations, too, on the company you have kept. Medical historians report many famous people who were arthritic. The poet Horace, Augustus Caesar and Cato the Censor are among your fellow sufferers. Lorenzo the Magnificent while still young in years became so undone by the disease that he is reported to have seemed old and decrepit. Henry IV of France suffered from pain in the joints of his jaws. Louis XIII was lame for several years, and Louis XIV had painful joints believed at the time to be caused by decaying teeth.

Famous soldiers in your company include Julius Caesar and Frederick the Great. Cardinal Richelieu, John Calvin, Lamartine, Chateaubriand, William Pitt, Rubens, La Rochefoucauld and Catherine di Medici all were arthritic at one time or another.

Because it is so old and widespread, rheumatism has long had its mythology. Sure cures for it have been offered since long before the first printed word, and it has been a source of income for charlatans. We no longer hear of wearing one's clothing backward as a cure, or of pulling the hair from the belly of a bear as it steps over the patient. But victims are still being offered special diets, miracle vibrators, "cosmic ray" generators and magic bracelets. Special investigators of the Federal Trade Commission and the Food and Drug Administration are kept busy protecting the public from gadgets and schemes dreamed up by those whose chief interest is in the patients' pocketbooks.

As the following chapters are read, it is hoped that they will point out why such things cannot succeed but why a proper outline of treatment can.

II What Are Arthritis and Rheumatism?

Before discussing the various forms of rheumatism, it would perhaps be well to review what is meant by some of the terms in common use. Doctors often speak a different language from layman and since this book is written by a doctor, but for laymen, agreement on the words to be used may be a good starting point. At present the most popular term is "arthritis." This comes from the Greek, *arthron*—joint; and *itis*—inflammation, and therefore literally means an inflamed joint. Although "arthritis" seems to be popularly used nowadays to describe any ache or pain in the entire skeleton, it should be reserved for cases of true joint involvement. On the other hand, physicians use the word "rheumatism" and the term "rheumatic diseases" as over-all designations to include painful conditions of the joints or their supports—capsules, ligaments, tendons and muscles. The French physician, Guillame de Baillou, is credited with introducing this word rheumatism early in the seventeenth century. The Greek root *rheum* means "to flow"—and was used because physicians in his day thought "noxious humors" (or vapors) flowed from one joint to another, causing the disease. In the later nineteenth century, as the "humoral" theory fell into disrepute, the term was used less and less by physicians, but remained in popular favor to designate indefinite muscular aches. Even today, when people hear the word rheumatism they are apt to think of the pain grandma had in her legs after sitting in a draft. But the American Rheumatism Association and its English counterpart, the Empire Rheumatism Council, now feel that this is the best general term for this whole group of diseases—hence we can correctly say that this manual discusses rheumatism or the rheumatic diseases. Likewise, "rheumatology" means the science or study of these conditions, a clinic devoted to their diagnosis and treatment is properly called a "rheumatology clinic," and a physician specializing in this field is a "rheumatologist."

True, the various forms of arthritis make up the largest and most important group of the rheumatic diseases, but also included is "fibrositis," in which the fibrous tissue in and around the joints is involved, rather than the joint itself; also, "psychogenic rheumatism" in which nervous or emotional reactions cause the patient to experience symptoms similar to those of arthritis, but without true joint changes; and even "neoplasms" (new growths) in which tumors invade the joint, either growing from the structures of the joint itself, or spreading to the joint from elsewhere.

Another term that perhaps should be defined is "peripheral joints," indicating all the joints of the upper and lower extremities: the shoulders, elbows, wrists, hands, fingers, hips, knees, ankles, feet and toes. These are distinct from the joints of the spinal column, and the jaws. Arthritis in the spine is called "spondylitis," *spondylo* meaning spine.

When we speak of the "physiology" of a joint (or indeed of tissue) we are referring to its day-to-day functions, including the normal action of blood vessels and nerves supplying it. The term "pathology" indicates an abnormality of the physiology. Thus, when we mention the "pathology of rheumatoid arthritis," or "the pathologic changes in rheumatoid arthritis," we are referring to the altered or abnormal physiology which finally makes an arthritic joint different from the normal.

A word frequently used as a synonym for joint is "articulation," and one may say "articulating surfaces," referring to the two ends of the bones that form the joint. It is interesting that this comes from the Latin *artus* meaning joint, whereas it will be recalled that "arthritis' is derived from the Greek word *arthron,* also meaning joint.

"Ankylosis" means stiffness, and an "ankylosed joint" there fore, is one that no longer moves. With partial ankylosis a joint still has some motion; a completely ankylosed joint is rigid.

Other new terms will be defined further on, in discussions of particular conditions.

III   What Does a Normal Joint Do?

Although this manual is not intended as a textbook of medicine, an understanding of certain basic pathologic changes will aid the patient in caring for himself. The facts presented are broad generalities, subject to extreme variations. The reader will realize that the human body, unlike a machine, does not always follow hard and fast rules, and that no two persons react exactly alike.

It may be helpful to consider first of all what makes up a normal joint and then to consider the changes caused by arthritis. Figure 1 represents a cross section of a joint. No joint in the body looks quite like this, but it shows the structures making up all the movable joints.

As can be seen, the ends of the bone are covered with car-

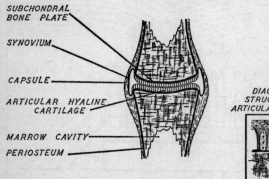

SUBCHONDRAL
BONE PLATE

SYNOVIUM

CAPSULE

ARTICULAR HYALINE
CARTILAGE

MARROW CAVITY

PERIOSTEUM

DIAGRAM OF
STRUCTURE OF
ARTICULAR CARTILAGE

NORMAL JOINT

FIGURE 1

tilage. That part in which the actual motion takes place is known as the articulating surface. Thus, bone never normally moves over bone; rather cartilage against cartilage. This cartilage is tough, elastic, and compressible, helping to absorb some of the shock of weight-bearing. It is a solid pad and has no blood vessels or nerves. It obtains its food by absorption from the tissue fluids in the joint. Between the articulating surfaces is the "joint space," the size exaggerated in these drawings. Actually, the joint space is quite narrow, and in weight-bearing joints, such as the knees, the space is only potential—for the weight of the body holds the articulating surfaces together. The synovium is a thin membrane forming the inner lining of the capsule and the outer lining of the joint. It secrets a small amount of fluid, keeping the normal joint constantly lubricated. Finally, the capsule which holds the joint together is made up of tough fibrous tissue continuous with the outer sheath of the bones, called the periosteum, from *peri*—around; and *osteum*—bone.

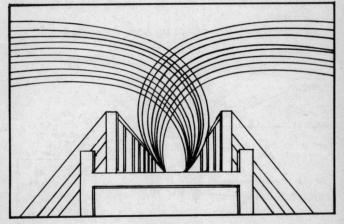

FIGURE 1A

Bridge under construction showing comparison to cartilage cell structure.

It is interesting to compare the structure of the cartilage cell, as shown in the enlarged diagram of Figure 1, with the structural steel framework of a modern bridge shown under construction in Figure 1A. Modern man has learned much about tensile strength from his own joints.

The primary function of any joint is motion. But not all joints move alike—each being designed for a particular task. Thus, a knee or an elbow is a hinge (Figure 2) type of joint; a shoulder or hip is a ball-and-socket type (Figure 3). The two bones of the forearm form a joint near the elbow in which one bone is round and turns in the socket of the other, while at the wrist one bone slides around the other (Figure 4), permitting the hand to be turned up (supinated) or down (pronated). In the spine, a sliding motion occurs. As the trunk is bent forward and

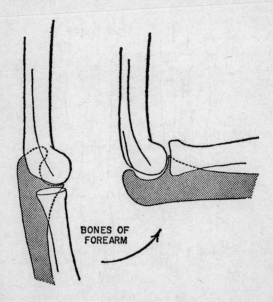

BONES OF
FOREARM

FIGURE 2

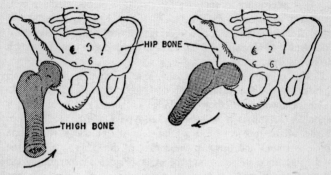

FIGURE 3

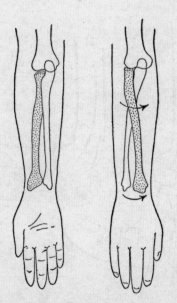

FIGURE 4

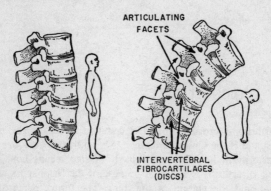

ARTICULATING FACETS

INTERVERTEBRAL FIBROCARTILAGES (DISCS)

FIGURE 5

backward, the articulating facets of any vertebra slide on the vertebra above and below (Figure 5). This construction also permits side-to-side bending as well as rotation of the spine.

Now, a joint moves because of muscular pull on the bones. And since these muscles are frequently connected to the outer part of the joint capsule, their contraction can influence the joint.

Different types of rheumatism alter these structures in different ways. A complete analysis of all changes in all types would fill a much larger volume than this one, but in succeeding chapters we shall try to consider the important changes in the more common types and show how these changes result in the symptoms peculiar to one or another.

IV Osteoarthritis

Osteoarthritis is probably the most common of all the rheumatic diseases and is the kind meant when it is said that "everyone gets some arthritis if he lives long enough." *Osteo* means bone, and this type of arthritis is so called because of the bony spurs which occur around the margin of the joint. The term "hypertrophic arthritis" is also used, and for a similar reason. *Hyper* means over, and *trophic,* growth. The little bony deposits are indeed overgrowths of calcium. A third term sometimes used is "degenerative joint disease," referring to the changes in the cartilage during this type of arthritis.

Figures 6, 7 and 8 give a composite representation of how the normal joint structures become altered. The first change is in the cartilage where the cells become swollen and edematous (filled with an abnormal amount of fluid). The cartilage then loses its dense homogeneous nature and shows a series of cracks called fibrillations. These resemble slightly the linear cracks seen in old marble columns and represent a degree of wear. Next, the cartilage shows signs of erosion. This starts as a flaking of the cartilage on its articular surface and may be only minor; or it may become so severe that the entire cartilage is eroded away. When this occurs, there is usually an abnormal strain at the outer margin of the bone where the ligaments and muscles are attached. Nature responds to this strain by the laying down of extra calcium. Bony spurs are thus produced much in the same manner as calluses and corns from the strain of a tight shoe. These spurs, or osteophytes, build up slowly over the years. They may be limited to the hands, where they usually first affect the end row of joints and are called "Heberden's nodes" after the

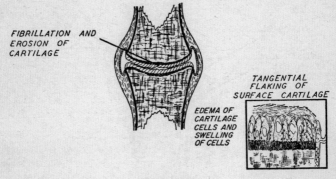

FIBRILLATION AND EROSION OF CARTILAGE

TANGENTIAL FLAKING OF SURFACE CARTILAGE

EDEMA OF CARTILAGE CELLS AND SWELLING OF CELLS

FIGURE 6

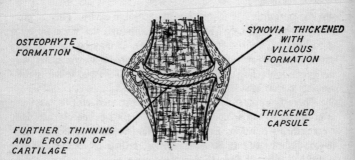

OSTEOPHYTE FORMATION

SYNOVIA THICKENED WITH VILLOUS FORMATION

THICKENED CAPSULE

FURTHER THINNING AND EROSION OF CARTILAGE

OSTEOARTHRITIS — ADVANCED

FIGURE 7

English physician, who in the 1700s first called attention to them. In many cases spurs become widespread, affecting almost all the joints, peripheral and spinal, even the jaws. As time goes on, these twin processes of cartilage-degeneration and osteophyte-formation may cause interference with the normal action of the joint. Usually, however, the changes progress to a moderate degree only and remain static for years. Occasionally, a sudden twist of a joint, or a blow, may break off one of the little osteo-

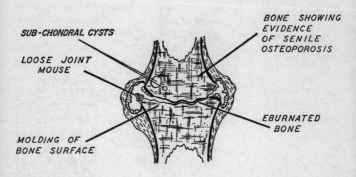

SUB-CHONDRAL CYSTS

BONE SHOWING
EVIDENCE
OF SENILE
OSTEOPOROSIS

LOOSE JOINT
MOUSE

EBURNATED
BONE

MOLDING OF
BONE SURFACE

FIGURE 8

phytes, permitting it to be free in the joint cavity. This is popularly referred to as a "joint mouse" although the scientific term is arthrolith (*arthro*—joint; *lith*—stone). It may be the size of a small piece of gravel. No harm comes unless it works its way between contacting surfaces, when it will cause much pain—similar to that of a large cinder in the eyelid—until it is dislodged.

There is apparently no single cause of osteoarthritis, as there is in diseases such as pneumonia, poliomyelitis or measles. Rather, osteoarthritis develops because of certain wearing processes within the joints, and it is sometimes described as "wear-and-tear arthritis." Not all the reasons that cause one person's joints to show signs of wear sooner than another's are entirely understood, but a few of them are. First, of course, is the matter of age—for osteoarthritis is rarely seen in people under 35, and is quite common in those over 65. Yet, this alone is not the final answer for many persons in their seventies have no symptoms of the condition and when their joints are x-rayed these show surprisingly few changes. Probably, just as important is the matter of heredity. As some families seem to show a tendency to heart disease or cancer, so others seem to have a tendency to develop osteoarthritis. Dr. Leon Sokoloff, pathologist at the National Institutes of Health, has shown that this is quite true in laboratory animals. Some of his strains of mice developed osteoarthritic changes at a comparatively early age; others almost never developed the condition. Then there can be repeated minor injuries to joints, "micro trauma." Piano players and typists sometimes develop changes in the end finger joints; pneumatic-drill operators, changes in the wrists; baseball and tennis players, changes in the shoulders. The Arabians, and others who stay for hours in a squatting position, may develop osteoarthritic knees. In addition to hereditary traits and continued minor traumas, impaired blood supply seems to be a cause. This type of arthritis has been produced experimentally in animals by narrowing the arteries supplying a joint to give only one-fourth as much blood as needed. The impaired nutrition then seems to help produce osteoarthritis. Other experiments have shown that laboratory animals will develop osteoarthritis more rapidly if fed a high-fat diet. Still others have indicated that osteoarthritis can be initiated by protecting weight bearing joints in the early formative years, thus depriving them of the strength-giving stress which comparable animals are permitted to obtain. Whether or not all these things are true in humans has not been determined. There are undoubtedly other influences not fully understood, possibly glandular imbalance or altered blood chemistry. Because the bony spurs in the region of the joints are composed of calcium, patients often suggest that an excessive intake of calcium may play a part. This, however, does not seem to be true. The trouble is not one of excessive calcium, but rather that the calcium, always circulating in the blood, is deposited in the wrong places.

Just as repeated minor injuries to the joint can produce osteoarthritis, so too, can a single severe injury. Such cases are spoken of as secondary osteoarthritis. Swelling of the cells and the resultant changes occur quite rapidly in contrast to the slow development of primary osteoarthritis. The baseball finger, which results from being hit on the end of a finger by a ball, is a secondary osteoarthritis; but the effect can be about the same as primary osteoarthritis in the end finger joints.

A curious fact which Dr. Robert Stecher in Cleveland discovered is that osteoarthritis of the fingers (Heberden's nodes), will not develop unless the nerve supply is intact. Thus, if a patient has suffered a stroke or other nerve damage, the nodes will develop only in the healthy fingers, not in the fingers of the paralyzed arm.

Symptoms: Surprisingly, persons having osteoarthritis do not always note their symptoms to be proportionate to the amount of change which has taken place. It is common for a routine x-ray to show extensive osteoarthritic changes in a person of sixty or sixty-five years suffering no pain. This is because neither the bony osteophytes nor the roughened cartilage is rich in pain-sensitive nerve endings. When pain is present it is usually from pressure on surrounding tissues or a temporary local inflammation. Knees, hips, and lower spine can be the most painful osteoarthritic joints, when there is a combination of thick roughened cartilage, pressure on surrounding tissues, and abnormal stress on ligaments and muscles. Stiffness is a common complaint of those who have osteoarthritis. It is noted particularily in the morning, after being in bed all night, or at other times after sitting a long time in one position, as at a movie or concert. The joints and surrounding tissues seem to "set" like jelly and must be limbered before sudden use. Cold, dampness, and fatigue increase this stiffness perceptibly, probably from interference with the blood supply to the joints and surrounding muscles.

Osteoarthritis is rarely disabling. It comes on insidiously, reaches a plateau and is likely to stay there for years, one of the unpleasant but rarely disastrous accompaniments of age. Since modern science does not yet know how to dissolve the calcium deposits or grow new cartilage, the condition cannot be cured in the sense that pneumonia or diphtheria is cured. However, since it is not the abnormal tissues so much as the inflammation around them that causes the symptoms, and the inflammation usually responds to treatment, the discomforts can be eased. Specific measures will be dealt with in the chapter on treatment, but persons with osteoarthritis must bear in mind that any strain to the joint—whether excessive use, exposure, or too much weight—can aggravate the condition; and anything that improves the circulation to the joint—heat, gentle massage, rest and exercise—should be helpful.

As I have said, osteoarthritis develops slowly. As the cartilage insidiously erodes and the bony spurs develop, the changes are so gradual that the surrounding tissues are able to accommodate themselves to the new growths. Thus considerable change may have taken place before the patient has any symptoms. Persons in the forty to fifty year group find they are unable to perform activities formerly done with ease and as the years go by they are aware that the affected joints are giving more persistent pain and stiffness. Occasionally the arthritic changes become so severe that a joint is hardly usable. This, fortunately, is rare.

At times, however, the symptoms may first be noted suddenly, after an accident. Then, the slowly developing spurs to which the tissues previously were accustomed seem to tear those tissues and initiate a painful chain of symptoms which may take some time to subside. Furthermore, pain may develop in other joints than those apparently injured. Thus, a person may twist his ankle stepping off a street car and find that not only the ankle is painful but the knee and hip as well.

Such cases sometimes have medico-legal importance. The injured person feels that the accident is the cause of his pain since he had no prior symptoms. The one responsible for the accident points out that there is evidence on the x-rays of changes which have been present for some years. What has happened, of course, is that the accident has caused a previously existing but quiescent arthritis to become symptomatic.

Any joint may be affected. The most common signs of osteoarthritis, especially in women, are the nodular enlargements of the end finger joints, which I have previously mentioned as being called Heberden's nodes. Often they are painless, but in extreme cases may be disabling. They are most likely to be severe in persons whose work requires much use of the fingers. Indeed, the disease shows itself in joints subject to excessive use or strain; consequently, people who are overweight may develop it in the knees, heavy laborers in the lower spine, and desk workers in the neck and upper part of the spine. And it shows up at times in unusual locations. A football player who played right guard for several years developed osteoarthritic changes in the joint where the collarbone meets the shoulder—from persistently bucking the line; a wrestler showed large spurs along his spine—the result of being slammed on the mat again and again; a seamstress developed a large node on the thimble finger; all unusual locations, but logical when one considers the cause.

Of considerable interest is the fact that osteoarthritis is usually limited to one joint or group of joints, as the fingers, the knees, or the hips. This would seem to throw cold water on the aging theory as a cause of arthritis for obviously one joint is as old as another in the same individual. Occasionally, however, the disease is widespread and is referred to as "primary generalized osteoarthritis." Another special form of osteoarthritis, which occurs particularly in women and apparently is strongly hereditary, affects not only the end row of finger joints but the middle row also. This type has been called "interphalangeal osteoarthritis." (The separate bones of the fingers are known as phalanges—plural of phalanx.) Persons so afflicted may have periods of considerable pain when individual joints are red, hot and swollen. As time goes on, sizeable nodules may develop on many of the finger joints, and some may be permanently stiffened. Persons so afflicted frequently have osteoarthritis in the neck, but rarely elsewhere.

V Rheumatoid Arthritis

Rheumatoid arthritis is the form of joint disease most widely publicized in recent years and is mainly responsible for the fact that arthritis is so feared. It can, indeed, produce serious joint troubles, even severe crippling. This, however, is far from being the usual outcome. Many cases are self-limiting, developing only occasionally into an acute attack, and many more do not go beyond a moderate degree of disability, without severe deformities.

Rheumatoid arthritis is so called because in the early stages it often resembles rheumatic fever (*oid* meaning like). It was formerly called either chronic infectious arthritis because infection was thought to be the cause, or atrophic arthritis, to describe the x-ray appearance of bone-wasting. Pathologists preferred the term proliferative arthritis, since this describes the increased size of the joints' lining membrane occurring in the disease. All of these synonyms for rheumatoid arthritis are gradually dropping out of use.

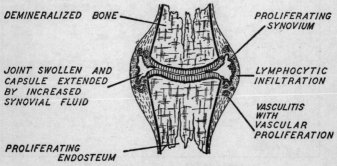

RHEUMATOID ARTHRITIS — EARLY

FIGURE 9

Whereas osteoarthritis, as described in the preceding chapter, is mainly a degenerative process occurring from the wear and tear of advancing years, rheumatoid arthritis is primarily an inflammatory condition which may occur at any age. This inflammation first manifests itself in the blood vessels supplying the synovium, and is referred to medically as a "vasculitis." (*Vasculum,* the Latin word for vessel, plus *itis*—inflammation.) As a result, the synovium (Figure 9) starts to thicken and proliferate (enlarge). Now, you will recall that we previously mentioned this

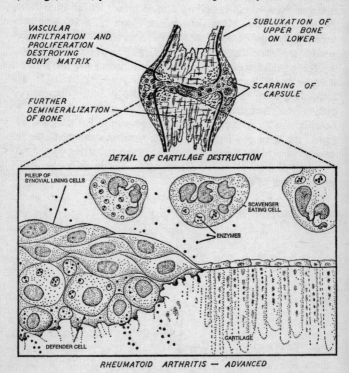

VASCULAR INFILTRATION AND PROLIFERATION DESTROYING BONY MATRIX

SUBLUXATION OF UPPER BONE ON LOWER

FURTHER DEMINERALIZATION OF BONE

SCARRING OF CAPSULE

DETAIL OF CARTILAGE DESTRUCTION

PILEUP OF SYNOVIAL LINING CELLS

SCAVENGER EATING CELL

ENZYMES

DEFENDER CELL

CARTILAGE

RHEUMATOID ARTHRITIS — ADVANCED

FIGURE 10

synovium as the thin membrane which generates the lubricating fluid of the joint. As it is stimulated by this "rheumatoid inflammation," it secretes more fluid, and the entire joint is therefore swollen. As the synovial growth increases it extends over the cartilage and may even form a thick, sticky, fibrous layer between the two cartilage surfaces. This is spoken of as "pannus formation." Now, if this inflammatory layer of synovial pannus persists any length of time, the cartilage with which it is in contact is destroyed (Figure 10). At the same time, the inflamed blood vessels in the ends of the bone are attacking the cartilage from beneath. As a result, extensive cartilagenous destruction may occur and bone may grow to bone forming an ankylosed (stiff) joint (Figure 11). However, this does not necessarily occur. The process may spontaneously stop, or be arrested by treatment at any point.

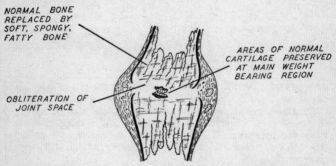

NORMAL BONE
REPLACED BY
SOFT, SPONGY,
FATTY BONE

AREAS OF NORMAL
CARTILAGE PRESERVED
AT MAIN WEIGHT
BEARING REGION

OBLITERATION OF
JOINT SPACE

RHEUMATOID ARTHRITIS WITH BONY ANKYLOSIS

FIGURE 11

Current thinking regarding the way inflammation affects a rheumatic joint has been well explained in The Arthritis Foundation's Annual Report for 1969 (© 1970 The Arthritis Foundation). It is quoted here, with its accompanying illustrations, by permission of the Foundation:

We now have, for the first time, a basic hypothesis about arthritis inflammation—about what causes it and how it operates. It is a hypothesis that makes rational sense. Many pieces of it have been confirmed. We know the targets for further research and controlled experiment.

The theory, and discoveries to back it up, point to abnormal events that happen in the tiny world and lives of certain cells of the body.

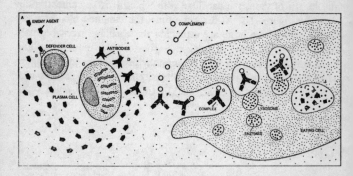

FIGURE 12

THE BODY'S NORMAL PROTECTION SYSTEM   Enemy agent (A) is contacted by defender blood cell (B) which gets "turned on" (C) and produces antibodies (D). Antibodies latch on to enemy agents (E), attract and join with complement (F). This triple complex is swallowed by eating cell (G) and brought in contact with lysosomes (H) which put their enzymes to work chewing up and digesting the complex (I and J).

THE BODY'S NORMAL PROTECTION SYSTEM

The first illustration shows the system by which the body normally deals with a foreign invader—an enemy agent (Figure 12).

An enemy agent can be a virus, a bacterium or something else that doesn't belong in the body and may threaten it with harm. Such an enemy, when it causes the body's defense system to react, is called an antigen.

When an antigen enters the body, it soon comes in contact with a defender cell, a type of blood cell called a lymphocyte.

Lymphocytes are "patrol" cells, a kind of police force. They circulate throughout the body. Under ordinary circumstances they possess an unerring ability to distinguish substances that are a proper and normal part of the body from substances that are foreign. They can tell "self" from "non-self." Their job is to spot enemy agents—antigens—and to do something about them.

When a lymphocyte comes in physical contact with an antigen, remarkable things happen. The lymphocyte cell is "turned on." It becomes transformed into a larger cell, then known as a plasma cell. This plasma cell sets about manufacturing antibodies—a militia called up specifically to strong-arm the particular invaders into submission. The antibodies thus manufactured have surfaces precisely keyed to fit surfaces of the antigens, so that the two can lock together.

As antibodies lock in with and immobilize antigens, a blood substance called complement is attracted and combines with them. The three-part combinations formed in this way are called complexes.

Now along comes a scavenger or "eating" cell, called a phagocytic cell, to perform a kind of sanitation service which

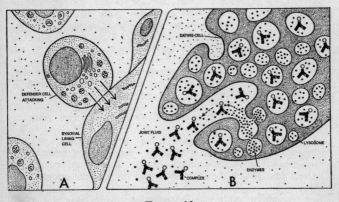

FIGURE 13

THE BODY ATTACKS ITSELF   Section A.   Confused defender cell attacks synovial lining cell of the joint.   Section B.   As complexes are gobbled in by eating cell, it becomes gorged. Powerful enzymes are vomited out and escape into surrounding joint fluid . . . where they seek out and damage joint tissue.

finishes the job. The eating cell forms an indentation in its surface and engulfs the complexes.

Inside the cell are little sacs (called lysosomes) containing powerful enzymes. The complexes and the sacs come together and the enzymes attack the complexes, break them up and "digest" them. This disposes of them and the threat to the body is thereby overcome.

THE BODY ATTACKS ITSELF

In arthritis, when the enemy agent appears on the scene in a human joint, strange things happen to this body protection system.

For one thing (and this is still partly theory), it appears that some defender cells, after they have been "turned on" and transformed by contact with the enemy antigen, become confused. Instead of making armies of antibodies, they themselves become agents of destruction. They move up against cells lining the joint where they pour out powerful substances that attack and damage the lining and cartilage. This is shown in Section A of Figure 13.

In Section B we see another kind of mishap that occurs in arthritis inflammation. Complexes—the bound combinations of enemy agent, antibody and complement—are swallowed up by eating cells, as they should be. But for some reason not yet understood, the complexes prove to be more than the eating cell can handle. Some of its enzymes escape from their sacs and the cell "vomits" them out into the surrounding fluid—the fluid of the joint. These enzymes are extremely potent substances, and they promptly attack and destroy cells of the joint lining and cartilage.

This inflammatory damage to joint tissues is arthritis.

Figure 10 illustrates how this inflammation attacks a joint.

One of the attacking agents is the "rain" of enzymes released by overfed eating cells (Section B of the second drawing). Another may be malfunctioning defender cells (lymphocytes) in actual contact with the joint tissue (Section A of the second drawing).

In addition, we see in the enlarged inset a mass of synovial lining cells and other cells which have multiplied and piled up in the area of attack. This jagged growth is called pannus. Substances bred in this mass eat into and damage the underlying cartilage.

Under this multiple attack the cartilage softens, weakens and ultimately can be destroyed completely.

Destruction of cartilage cells throws off an assortment of substances and debris. New eating cells rush into the joint area to clean up this biological trash. Some new lymphocytes may attack cartilage by mistake. And some of the new eating cells spew out their enzymes as the first ones did, thus pouring still more enzymes into the area of inflammation.

Thus, once triggered by an as-yet-unidentified agent (virus-?), arthritis inflammation can to some extent be self-reinforcing and self-perpetuating.

A trigger virus itself might also add to the holocaust by continuing to disrupt the function of eating cells, which in turn release still more destructive enzymes.

So inflammation increases, the disease progresses, pannus continues to pile up, and in time joint cartilage disappears.

For the human victim of arthritis, the result is ever-increasing suffering and pain and encroaching disability.

The exact cause of rheumatoid arthritis is not known. Indeed, there may not be any single cause. It seems possible that a combination of circumstances may be necessary. One of the oldest and still widely held views is that this form of arthritis is the result of an infection; but to date, no infectious agent has been isolated or proved. Investigators continue to try to discover whether it is a bacterium, a virus, or some organism that may have properties of each of these. It seems possible that the organism would not have to invade the joint itself to produce arthritis. Rather, the joint changes may be due to toxic or allergic influences from infection elsewhere in the body. Changes in the glandular secretions of the body may also play a part, or there may be a deficiency in some of the minerals in the blood stream. Vitamin deficiencies have also been suspected; however, a rather thorough investigation of all of the known vitamins has not shown any significant alteration in these. Emotional upset and nervous strain, while probably not a basic cause, can weaken the patient and reduce the natural resistance of the body. In this same category are persistent physical strain and general debility, continued exposure to damp and cold, and local injury to joints. All these serve to weaken the human organism and make it less resistant to arthritis.

There is some rather interesting evidence to indicate that patients with rheumatoid arthritis react against some of their own tissues and many physicians therefore feel that rheumatoid arthritis is a disease of "auto-immunity." To explain what is meant by this, we shall have to digress a moment from our discussion of arthritis. Most people have read that it is impossible under normal circumstances to graft (or transfer) any of the body's organs from one person to another except in the case of identical twins. This is due to the complex protective or immune mechanism with which we are born. So when a heart or kidney is to be transplanted, the person receiving the new organ must take large doses of drugs which suppress the immune reaction. And one of the hazards of such operations is the susceptibility to infection brought about by this change in the normal immune function. However, it is known that the immune mechanism can get out of kilter. A Japanese physician by the name of Hakaru Hashimoto demonstrated this in the case of people who for unknown reasons become sensitive to their own thyroid secretion. The condition has been named "Hashimoto's thyroiditis." So, too, there is some evidence that a rheumatoid patient is reacting against some of his own tissues. There are, however, many gaps in this theory and it is far from proved.

A puzzling influence to be reckoned with as a cause of arthritis is heredity. When large groups of patients are studied it will be found that many are from families where there are other cases of the disease. Occasionally one finds families in which a surprising number are afflicted. I have treated a family in which the mother and two daughters were arthritics. In other cases studied there have been not only brothers and sisters but cousins, aunts and uncles. But several years ago when a research team from the National Institutes of Health made a detailed study of this situation, it concluded that such instances were no more than coincidental. Their investigators felt that no scientific evidence exists to indicate rheumatoid arthritis is inherited.

Symptoms: Rheumatoid arthritis may appear in a variety of ways. Indeed, its onset is so varied that it is difficult to describe a typical case. As in rheumatic fever, the symptoms may come abruptly. A person may awaken in the morning with the wrist painful and tender, and then by noontime the joint may be hot and swollen. The joint may remain in this condition for several days and then subside, with similar symptoms in another joint, say, a knee. A few days later an elbow and a wrist may both be involved. This "migratory polyarthritis" may continue for weeks, with the symptoms eventually settling into one or two joints and staying there for many weeks or even months. Often, however, after the acute phase has passed, the joints are once more entirely normal. Months or years later the same process may be repeated, with perhaps permanent joint damage.

More commonly the symptoms come on gradually. The patient notes soreness and stiffness or swelling in one joint for several weeks. As time goes on, the acute swelling is replaced by permanent enlargement. Over the years other joints become similarly involved, and later every joint in the body may show changes. The fingers and toes are quite commonly involved. Indeed, when the fingers are not involved fairly early, the diagnosis is always somewhat questionable. Oddly, rheumatoid arthritis usually singles out the middle joints; osteoarthritis usually develops first in the end joints (Heberden's nodes).

If the disease progresses, any combination of joints may be involved. Owing to the destruction of cartilage, various deformities may be produced, and some joints may become stiff. Since the joints are tender and painful, patients have a tendency to hold them in the position most comfortable. This alone can cause development of deformities. Such a condition is frequently seen in the knees after a patient has put pillows under them during the acute phase. Later, it is found that they cannot be completely extended. Each knee is a little bent and as the patient again starts to walk, the weight of the body bends it further. These "flexion deformities" may be hard to correct; indeed, some require surgical help.

So much has been said and written about the deformity of joints in rheumatoid arthritis that many physicians and laymen alike get the impression that these are inevitable. This is not true. All disease processes vary. In an epidemic of scarlet fever one child may die, and another have only a slight rash. So, too, in rheumatoid arthritis any course is possible—but most cases are mild to moderate, with no crippling deformities.

Although the joint indications of rheumatoid arthritis are the most dramatic, they are not the only changes. It is a systemic disease, and the vasculitis which was previously described can occur in any organ in the body. Muscular symptoms are quite frequent and may involve muscle groups which are quite far distant from the particular joints involved. Thus, it is not uncommon for patients with swollen knees and feet to develop sore neck muscles, or sore chest muscles, as well as sore leg muscles. In addition to the soreness there may be marked weakness and extreme fatigue. And as the disease progresses muscular wasting may occur. Many patients find that the early morning hours, just after awakening, are their worst. Getting out of bed they are "stiff all over" and may not limber up for two to three hours. This "morning stiffness" which affects particularly the hands led Dr. Philip Hench, the discoverer of cortisone, to describe rheumatoid arthritics as belonging to "The Order of the Dripping Washcloth." It is commonly necessary to run warm water over the hands before the face can be washed or shaved.

In the acute stages there may be fever, weakness and even extreme prostration. Anemia may be persistent and troublesome. Later, the heart may be involved, the lungs, or the kidneys, even the eyes. The vasculitis may invade the nerves, causing numbness, tingling and burning. It is truly a variable and capricious disease.

Although it most commonly starts about the age of twenty-four or twenty-five, it can begin at any age; the author has treated a child of three and a woman of eighty-four for their first attacks. Both sexes are involved, but for some reason that is still not known, women outnumber men three or four to one. Rheumatoid arthritis has been found among all races and in all climates and in all countries. It is indeed a universal scourge.

VI Arthritis of the Spine

Two major forms of arthritis affect the spine. One is a degenerative type and occurs in persons over 50 years of age. The other type is an inflammatory type and always starts before the age of 35.

The degenerative type corresponds to osteoarthritis found elsewhere. Symptoms come gradually, showing first stiffness and soreness; pain that comes later is seldom severe; but the osteoarthritic spurs may build up in areas where nerves branch off from the spinal cord. In such cases, symptoms will be noted in regions quite distant from the spine itself. I recall two dentists with similar complaints. They were having increasing difficulty holding the dental drill more than a few minutes. Only after releasing the drill and exercising the hands under warm water were they able to get rid of the dead feeling in the hands. Each thought he had some arthritis of the hand, yet, neither did. The trouble was osteoarthritis in the neck. Then, we have seen many patients who awaken with pain in the back of the head and upper portion of the neck when they sleep with the neck twisted. There, too, nerves branching off from the spinal cord were irritated by osteoarthritic spurs.

In the inflammatory type of spinal arthritis, changes take place in the joints of the spine which are very much like those described as occurring in rheumatoid arthritis. For this reason, it was formerly called rheumatoid arthritis of the spine or rheumatoid spondylitis (*spondylo*—spine). But changes between the two diseases are so marked that it now seems better to catalog them separately; and the term ankylosing spondylitis (*ankylose*-stiff) is now the official designation. Physicians of a generation ago usually called it Marie-Strümpell disease. The French physician Pierre Marie, and the German physician Ernst Adolph Gottfried von Strümpell, were the first to study and describe the condition accurately, and their work during the latter years of the nineteenth century led later physicians to name the condition after them.

Although ankylosing spondylitis may come abruptly, with acute generalized backache and symptoms of fever, malaise, and weakness, an insidious onset is more common. More than three-quarters of all cases start in the lower spine, and there are almost ten male cases to one female. The most common age of onset is between twenty and thirty. Thus, it is primarily a disease of the young male adult. Persistent low backache is probably the most common early symptom. About one-tenth of all cases start as recurring attacks of sciatica. Indefinite pains through the muscles of the legs may also precede an attack. In those few cases which start in the upper spine or neck, there may be unusual and bizarre symptoms. Abdominal pain imitating gall bladder disease, or chest pain imitating pleurisy or a heart attack, may be the initial complaint owing to the inflammatory condition in the spine pressing on the nerves which go to these organs. As the disease progresses, the pain varies according to the individual, severe in some, mild in others; in many it is cyclical, alternating between periods of severe pain and others of relative freedom.

The most distinguishing characteristic of this form of spinal arthritis, however, is gradually increasing stiffness. This may first be noted only as difficulty in leaning forward. Later there may be trouble bending over to put on the socks or to tie the shoes. In extreme cases this may progress to a completely rigid back, the so-called "poker spine." As the condition affects the upper spine there is a tendency for the spine to pull forward, producing a hunching effect.

Ankylosing spondylitis is an extremely variable and unpredictable disease. It may confine itself only to the sacroiliac joints in the pelvis or it may involve the entire spine, including the neck. About one-fourth of the cases will have arthritis of the joints outside the spine. When present, it resembles the peripheral rheumatoid arthritis previously described. There is, however, a tendency to involve large joints such as the shoulders, hips, knees, and ankles, rather than the small joints of the fingers or feet. It is of considerable interest, too, that eye complications and heart involvement are more frequent in this form of arthritis than in any other (but still occur in a minority of patients).

In ankylosing spondylitis more than any other rheumatic disease (except perhaps gout), the patient's future depends on how actively he pursues his home treatments. Just what he should do depends on his physician's instructions—how to do it will be found later in this manual.

VII Miscellaneous Rheumatic Conditions

FIBROSITIS

In contrast to those types of rheumatism in which the joint structures themselves are involved and which therefore constitute a true arthritis, another common rheumatic disease in fibrositis. As the name implies, this is an inflammation in the fibrous connective tissue rather than in the joints. This tissue is general throughout the body, linking together the various muscles, tendons, and even the joint capsules. If one were to examine under a microscope a section of muscle from a case of fibrositis, it would be seen that the connective tissue fibers are swollen and infiltrated with small blood cells. However, as the cartilage and synovial lining of the joint are not affected, alterations in the size and shape of the joint do not occur. At times fibrositis may be a forerunner of true rheumatoid arthritis. Frequently, however, it is separate, persisting for years without other involvement. An extremely painful form of fibrositis occurring particularly in people over 50 years of age is called "Polymyalgia rheumatica." This usually responds to a short course of steroid therapy.

Although the exact cause of fibrositis is not known, it seems probable that it is basically due to infection. Probably a variety of infections may touch off the condition. For example, the most common variety of fibrositis is the lumbago that often accompanies grippe or flu. Acute though it is, this usually clears up when the underlying condition improves. At times, however, the infection either persists or else causes changes in the fibrous connective tissue that continue until one has a chronic generalized ailment.

Symptoms: The most characteristic form of chronic fibrositis is rather cyclic, recurring at intervals of months or even years, persisting for a while and gradually clearing only to recur. A generalized ache, rather than true pain, is a common complaint, and patients frequently say it is "just like a toothache," to describe how the muscles of the arms or legs feel. Fibrositis occurs more often in the neck region than elsewhere, and in the chest muscles between the ribs. There it may be confused with heart pain or with pleurisy. Symptoms are usually most noticeable in the morning when the patient first arises. He may find difficulty getting out of bed and need time to limber up. The hands may feel tight and stiff as if swollen. There may be mild swelling of the fingers making it difficult to put on the rings. As the hands become limber, this swelling disappears. Patients then get along well enough through the day but are fatigued by evening. Their symptoms are likely to be accentuated during cold, damp, rainy weather, when they are overtired or under emotional stress.

RUPTURED INTERVERTEBRAL DISC

The vertebrae forming the backbone are separated from one another by pads of disc-like cartilage—the "intervertebral cartilages" (Figure 14). These are composed of a thick outer layer of tough fibrous tissue and a small, soft, sponge-like center or core, called the nucleus. When one bends forward the motion squeezes together the front and extends the rear of the intervertebral discs (Figure 5). The disc obviously must be elastic. If subject to great stress and strain, as might occur from a sudden stretch, or from the compressing action of a sudden fall, the outer fibrous layer of the disc may be torn and the spongy center nucleus forced out (Figure 14). This tearing usually occurs at the rear of the disc and since the spinal cord lies in the canal just behind the vertebrae, the protruding material may press on the spinal cord, irritating it and causing symptoms of pain over the region supplied

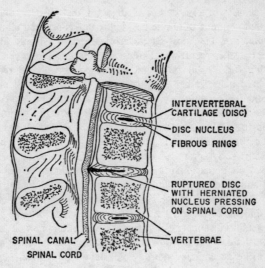

INTERVERTEBRAL
CARTILAGE (DISC)

DISC NUCLEUS

FIBROUS RINGS

RUPTURED DISC
WITH HERNIATED
NUCLEUS PRESSING
ON SPINAL CORD

SPINAL CANAL   VERTEBRAE
SPINAL CORD

FIGURE 14

by the nerve irritated. Usually there is a small local hemorrhage
with inflammation. As time goes on, this may be absorbed and
although the disc nucleus still protrudes, pressure on the cord
subsides and symptoms are relieved. If there should be another
strain, further hemorrhage may cause further swelling with re-
newal of symptoms. This process may be repeated many times.

Symptoms: The most significant symptom of ruptured intervertebral disc is severe pain in the back—most often in the lower
back, and usually radiating into a leg; but sometimes in the neck,
radiating into an arm. It is usually initiated by some injury, although this is not always the case. The pain may be severe enough
to incapacitate the patient, making even his turning over in bed
painful. After a few weeks the condition may be completely relieved, and the patient remain symptom-free. It appears that at
least half of all the cases of ruptured intervertebral disc have a
single severe attack with no recurrence. The other half, however,

have the same trouble again, at varying intervals, usually after an injury or an accident. The severity of the attacks may differ, some completely incapacitating the patient and others causing only a moderate degree of persistent backache. Now and then a case progresses to the extent that weakness of a leg with a wasting of the muscles develops. Although the lower (lumbar) spine is the most common place for this condition, nevertheless it can occur anywhere along the spine. Pain is always a prominent symptom; but the location and extent of the pain radiation depends on the particular disc which is ruptured. If in the lower spine, it may be hard to distinguish from ankylosing spondylitis. When it is in the neck region patients may complain of severe pain on any motion of the neck, with symptoms of numbness and tingling in the arms and hands similar to osteoarthritis. Indeed, many cases of osteoarthritis in the neck region are accompanied by a bulging or a protrusion of the disc without actual rupture, but prominent enough to press on the spinal cord and give symptoms.

An accurate diagnosis of ruptured intervertebral disc is not always easy. It may be confused with a sprained back or with arthritis of the spine. Yet, differentiation is important, for in severe cases only removal of the torn disc will bring about relief from the painful symptoms experienced. A study of the patient's reflexes and skin sensitivity may be helpful. If the disc has been ruptured for some time, the weight of the body usually forces the vertebrae on either side of the injured disc closer together. This can be seen in a routine x-ray. However, the disc itself is not visible since it is not dense enough to stop x-rays and cast its shadow on the film. To clinch the diagnosis a "myelogram" is usually done. This consists of injecting into the spinal canal an iodized oil which can be visualized by x-ray. The patient is placed on a tilt table, and as his position is varied, the flow of the iodized oil can be followed. Normally, the flow is smooth from one end of the canal to the other but if a disc is ruptured and protruding into the canal the oil will be blocked and its flow stalled at such a point. The surgeon will, therefore, know where to operate to remove the protruding disc.

STRAINS AND SPRAINS

These conditions are frequent in the muscles and joints. When a joint is sprained, the strong nonelastic ligaments that bind the bones together are torn because they are stretched beyond their capacity. That brings on a hemorrhage into the tissues, causing the joint to be swollen and tender. Healing takes place slowly, as the hemorrhage is absorbed. About the same condition occurs in muscle strains, where a muscle is stretched too much. Relief comes as the blood is slowly absorbed. Either a sprain or a strain may cause a scar in a ligament or muscle, making a weakened area. Sprains of the knee are frequently accompanied by a tearing of the cartilage at the joint surface, where a further complication may be a locking of the joint. Sprains of the back muscles usually occur in the lower spine, being brought on by attempts to lift objects beyond the patient's strength.

WHIPLASH INJURIES

This term is commonly used by almost everyone today, physicians and laymen. Yet, many legal authorities have strongly condemned it as being vague and inaccurate. "Cervical sprain" or "sprain of the cervical spine tissues" has been recommended as being more descriptive. Yet, the term persists and will be used in this paragraph. As almost everyone now knows these conditions are usually the result of injuries sustained in an automobile accident. Either the patient was a passenger in a car traveling at fairly high speeds when it collided with another vehicle, or else the patient was sitting in a stopped car which was struck forcibly from behind by a moving car or truck. In either case, the sudden change in position causes the head to snap first in one direction and then in the other. As a result, there is a tearing of ligaments and tendons with resultant pain. No bones are broken or dislocated, but the pain may persist for weeks or even months. Unfortunately, there is no accurate way to measure the exact amount of damage. Patients often continue to complain of pain long after healing of the sprained structures should have taken place. Because there is no laboratory test which can tell exactly how much tissue has been torn or just when it has healed, the legal ramifications of whiplash injuries are often rather complicated.

PSYCHOGENIC RHEUMATISM

Psychogenic rheumatism is the condition in which pain is experienced in the joints or their surrounding tissues not as a result of organic abnormalities in the joints but instead, from emotional causes. It may at times be difficult to distinguish psychogenic rheumatism from true arthritis, or from fibrositis, but it is well to know which it is for the methods of treatment are different. As mentioned, the cause of psychogenic rheumatism does not lie in the joints but in the emotional make-up of the patient.

True arthritis, however, may also be influenced by emotional upsets. This can even happen to fairly stable persons if exposed to long periods of unusual emotional tension. Take, for example, the wife who nurses a paralytic husband in the face of a much-reduced family income; or the woman who must raise a family with a husband who drinks too much. A person may withstand such a stress for years until resistance finally collapses and true arthritis develops.

Psychogenic rheumatism, however, is something different. Instead of occurring in a formerly stable person who has undergone severe emotional tension, it hits the emotionally unstable who are easily upset by minor stress. Frequently the trouble comes from the inability of the patient to cope with even the everyday issues of life. Instead of meeting the issues, admitting a defeat from time to time, and then resolutely trying again, he retreats behind his "arthritis." Sometimes the "arthritis" is used as an attention-getter or as an attention-holder. Sometimes the "arthritis" becomes a "way of life"—a poor solution for what appears to be an insoluble conflict. None of this is conscious, and the pain is just as real as it is in true organic arthritis. The patient does not just imagine he has pain; he actually has it, but it is due to the subconscious working of the mind and not to changes within the joints. This is a difficult concept for patients to appreciate. It is covered in more detail in another chapter.

RHEUMATIC FEVER

Rheumatic fever holds a unique place in this group of diseases, for its chief danger is injury to the heart rather than to the joints. In the acute phase, numerous joints may be red, hot, swollen, painful and tender. The process may migrate from joint to joint, with one of them clearing and another becoming affected. It is often spoken of as an "acute migratory polyarthritis." The acute symptoms may persist for months, but when this phase is over, the joints nearly always heal completely. On the other hand, the heart itself may be damaged permanently and rheumatic fever in children accounts for many cases of chronic heart disease in adults. It will be recalled that in rheumatoid arthritis the reverse is true, with the joints finally showing permanent damage and the heart usually remaining unchanged.

BURSITIS

Although bursitis is usually an acute condition and may last only a week, those who have had an attack are not likely to forget it. The sudden onset of severe pain, so intense at times as to require narcotics for relief, is something the sufferer is bound to remember. Yet this term, "bursitis," which has become so common with doctors as well as laymen, is not entirely accurate. Furthermore, although the shoulder is the most usual place affected, it is not the only one. To understand all this, one must understand something about a bursa—what it is and what it does. It will be recalled that in Chapter III, the diagram of the normal joint showed a structure called the synovial membrane, which, it was pointed out, generates a lubricating fluid. In the small joints of the fingers and toes the fluid lubricant produced by this synovium is sufficient for their operation. But larger joints need more than this, and it is here that the bursa plays its part. For a bursa is a small sac located near a joint and connected to it by a thin tubular duct. As the joint moves, it stimulates the bursa to generate a lubricating fluid which is carried through the duct and in the joint supplements the synovial fluid. Large joints such as the hips and shoulders have several bursae (plural of bursa) which may be called on for increased "oil" when the joints are used extensively.

Now, the largest bursa at the shoulder is located near the outer tip of that joint. Passing over it is a strong tendon which helps to rotate the arm (the supraspinatus tendon, so called because the muscle from which it originates is located above the spine of the shoulder blade) and over that tendon is a bony ridge which forms part of the shoulder joint. Because of this bony ridge, the tendon at this point is quite susceptible to injury. Often, after a tendon is injured, calcium will be deposited by the blood at the point of injury as part of the healing process. This calcium deposit may vary from a tiny amount the size of a pinhead, to a large amount the size of a lima bean. Occasionally multiple deposits occur.

Inflammation around one of these calcium deposits causes the severe pain mentioned at the beginning of this discussion. The bursa which is underneath the tendon is only secondarily affected. This is why most doctors now refer to this condition as "calcific (or calcareous) tendinitis." The distinction, however, is a fine one, for it seems improbable that one structure is involved without the other. Just why this inflammation should occur is not always clear. Sometimes it is started by a new injury to the tendon, as might happen after a game of tennis, or bowling, or after polishing a car, or painting a room. But other attacks come on without any evident cause—some even starting in the middle of the night and awakening the patient from a sound sleep.

The acute phase of calcific tendinitis may last from one or two days to two or three weeks. During this period the pain may continue to be severe. Since it is increased on motions of the shoulder, the patient keeps his arm locked tightly at the side. The area overlying the calcific deposit is extremely tender and the patient therefore guards his shoulder against any contact.

When this painful phase of calcific tendinitis subsides, relief is usually complete. But in some cases a dull ache persists, increased on certain motions of the arm. This is known as "chronic bursitis," or "chronic calcific tendinitis."

So far as treatment is concerned, no one mode of therapy has proved of benefit in all cases. X-ray radiation, diathermy applications, ultrasonic soundings, novocain and hydrocortisone injections, and oral phenylbutazone have all proved effective in some cases and all have failed in others. It may at times be necessary to try several forms of treatment successively or in combination before relief is obtained. In some of the chronic cases (and indeed in some of the acute cases) surgical removal of the calcium may be necessary.

BICIPITAL TENDINITIS AND ADHESIVE CAPSULITIS

These are two conditions which may also cause pain in the shoulder. At times either may be confused with calcific tendinitis. The bicipital tendon (so called because it runs in a groove between two bony ridges) is situated at the front part of the shoulder. It forms one of the upper attachments of the biceps muscle (that muscle which flexes the forearm, and is the delight of strong-arm "muscle men"). When it becomes irritated or inflamed it too causes pain in the shoulder. In this case, however, the pain is usually more moderate and of more gradual onset, but apt to persist longer than in calcific tendinitis. Both conditions, but particularly bicipital tendinitis, may give rise to a generalized inflammation of the shoulder capsule. When this occurs, the inner lining of the capsule becomes sticky like adhesive tape and it is therefore called adhesive capsulitis. These adhesions cause more and more restriction of the shoulder motion, and in time it may be impossible to raise the arm from a position tight against the body. It is then called a "frozen shoulder." Once this condition has developed, surgical correction may be necessary. Usually, however, it can be prevented by active physical therapy and injections of hydrocortisone into the joint.

OTHER FORMS OF BURSITIS

When a bursa is injured, it usually responds by an increase in its fluid production. The best known example of this is "water on the knee" which occurs when the main bursa supplying the knee is struck. Constant mild irritation of a bursa may cause it to thicken and enlarge gradually, causing a lump which, when felt, resembles a large callus. "Housemaid's knee" and "bartender's elbow" are examples.

EPICONDYLITIS

The muscles which help rotate the forearm are attached to bony prominences on either side of the elbow joint. These points are known as the epicondyles (*epi*—upon; *condyle*—a knuckle). If there is a sprain or tear at this point of attachment, an inflammation occurs known as epicondylitis. Tennis players are particularly susceptible to this because the motion used in swinging a tennis racket will, at times, cause such a sprain or tear. The pain usually comes on quite abruptly and the player frequently is aware of the instant in which the tear occurs. At other times, it may come on more gradually during the twenty-four hours following a rather strenuous game. Most cases last only a few days and quiet down spontaneously but others may persist for weeks and be disabling. A rather prominent player developed epicondylitis while practicing for a national tournament. Not only did he miss the tournament, but when pain persisted in spite of conservative treatment, it was necessary to apply a cast and keep the elbow immobile for six weeks. Fortunately, such severe cases are rare.

ALLERGIC JOINT REACTIONS

Occasionally joints will be involved in a generalized allergic reaction. This is most common following an injection of some substance to which the individual is sensitive—such as penicillin or tetanus antitoxin. One joint, or several, will swell rather abruptly and remain so for several days. Despite rather prominent enlargement there is no pain, only a feeling of tightness. The diagnosis at first may be confusing, but the cause is usually apparent from other allergic manifestations, particularly giant itching hives. It usually responds promptly to antihistamines, though large doses may be necessary.

NEOPLASMS (New Growths)

Fortunately, tumors of the joints are rare. They may arise from the various structures within the joint itself (synovium and cartilage) or they may form in the muscle or bone outside the joint and invade it secondarily. When they are found, surgical removal is usually indicated.

TRAUMATIC ARTHRITIS

A joint that has been injured usually responds in one of two ways, depending on the type of injury. If there has been a direct blow, the synovial membrane will be injured and increase its secretion. The joint will then be swollen. When this occurs in the knee, it is commonly referred to as "water on the knee." The extent and duration of the swelling will depend on the severity of the blow. If the joint has suffered a compressing type of injury as happens when a baseball is "caught" on the end of the finger, the cartilage is damaged, and may even be split. At the same time there will be some injury to the synovium with resultant swelling of the joint, usually less than in a direct blow. In either case, however, osteophytes are apt to develop and a "secondary" osteoarthritis follows. When this is fully developed it is usually indistinguishable from "primary" osteoarthritis described in chapter IV.

PALINDROMIC ARTHRITIS

In the rare, yet interesting, condition called palindromic arthritis, there is a recurring acute swelling of one or several joints. This swelling develops rather suddenly and the joint or joints affected are warm, red and tender. The condition lasts from two to three days and then subsides. Attacks may recur at irregular intervals, usually two to three months apart. Usually there is no residual damage to any joint. Some cases, however, develop into true rheumatoid arthritis. Others are apparently allergic in origin and may be relieved by histamine desensitization. Others seem to be non-specific and may continue to recur for ten or twenty years without significant change in the pattern. It is this feature which has given the condition its name, "palindromic," meaning recurrent, or repeating the course.

SEPTIC ARTHRITIS

This is the term applied to a joint when it is the seat of infection. Such joins usually are acutely inflamed. They are very painful and quite tender. If uncontrolled, the infection may cause rapid destruction of the joint and eventual stiffening. Infection can enter a joint in one of two ways. It may be introduced directly—as would happen in an accident when infected material is driven into the joint; or it may also be carried to the joint through the blood stream from a "focus" somewhere else. Tuberculous arthritis is sometimes an exception to the rule that all septic joints are acutely swollen and painful. In contrast to the symptoms presented when a joint is infected by a streptococcus or a staphylococcus, one infected by tuberculosis may develop quite slowly and be much less intense. If untreated, however, the joint will still eventually be destroyed. Cases of septic arthritis usually respond to treatment with the appropriate antibiotic. This may at times be given directly into the joint as well as by mouth or intramuscularly.

"THE COLLAGEN DISEASES"

This manual would not be complete without a short mention of a group of diseases, which, although not entirely understood, are quite important. Although the diseases are unrelated in many ways, they are grouped together for the purpose of convenience under the general heading of "collagen diseases" because of the fact that in each of them certain fibers in the connective tissue— called collagen fibers—seem to be primarily affected, either themselves or the glue-like mucus that holds them together. These are the fibers which actually bind the muscles, tendons and joint capsules together. Then, too, another characteristic which all these diseases have in common is their long unpronounceable names. The first is known as systemic (or disseminated) lupus erythematosus, sometimes shortened to its initals, S. L. E. or L. E. In this disease, joint symptoms often identical with those of rheumatoid arthritis may be noted. Indeed, in some cases it may be impossible to separate the two diseases, and many investigators feel that they are different phases of the same basic disease. On the other hand, cases of systemic lupus erythematosus, not infrequently develop involvement of vital organs such as the lungs, heart, kidneys and liver. Skin changes, too, are frequent and one of the most characteristic is a red blush over the nose and cheek, spoken of as a "butterfly rash." It is not uncommon to see a case of systemic lupus start with joint symptoms closely mimicking those of rheumatoid arthritis. As time goes on, however, these may subside completely to be replaced by symptoms from the affected organs. Young women under thirty years of age are particularly prone to it.

The next of the collagen diseases is known as polyarteritis (or periarteritis) nodosa, because small knots form as a result of inflammation around the arteries (*poly*—many; *peri*—around). These microscopic nodes forming around the tiny little blood vessels finally obstruct them completely, leading to impairment of the nutrition of the tissue supplied. The process can take place in any part of the body; in the muscle, or within the joint, or in any of the various organs. It may be rather localized or it may be quite widespread. Symptoms depend entirely on the location of the blood vessels that are obstructed.

The third collagen disease is called scleroderma (*sclero*—hard; *derma*—skin). In this condition the skin loses its pliability and elasticity and becomes hardened almost like leather. The condition usually starts in the arms and then develops in the legs. It may finally extend to involve the face and eventually the skin over the trunk. Sclerotic (hard) changes may also be taking place internally, particularly in the lungs and in the esophagus. And because the condition may thus progress to various areas in the body, it is now usually called "progressive systemic sclerosis."

The final disease in this group is called dermatomyositis (*derma*—skin; *myo*—muscles; *itis*—inflammation). This condition usually starts off with a rash and some watery swelling in the skin, to be followed by generalized weakness, loss of weight, fatigue, fever and extreme stiffness. It may be accompanied by deposits of calcium through the tendon, skin and muscle. Only rarely are the joints involved. When only the muscles are involved the condition is called "polymyositis." A curious fact is that the muscles of the upper arms and upper legs are the ones most seriously affected while those below the elbows and knees often remain normal. Because of this, patients have considerable difficulty combing their hair—or getting up from a sitting position. The disease is subject to remissions and recurrences but is apt to be quite chronic. Many cases respond dramatically to the steroid drugs, others are singularly resistant to treatment.

CHONDROCALCINOSIS

In this condition, calcium is deposited in the joint cartilages leading to a distinctive x-ray appearance (*chondro*—cartilage; *osis*—a condition). It is characterized by repeated attacks in which a particular joint will suddenly become swollen, painful, warm and tender. It thus, may resemble gout (discussed in the second half of this book) and the disease has been called "pseudo-gout."

The attack may last only a few days or several weeks. Any joint in the body may be involved, but the knees suffer most frequently. In occasional cases, the calcified cartilages may seriously impair the function of the involved joints.

REITER'S SYNDROME

This condition—named for the German physician who described it in 1916—is characterized by joint symptoms which may suggest rheumatoid arthritis. But with the arthritis, there is also acute inflammation in the eyes and genital organs or lower bowel. It occurs predominantly in men—and most frequently in military installations or camps. Although the condition can be exceedingly severe, the prognosis for eventual recovery is good. It seems quite probable that Reiter's Syndrome is due to an infection.

VIII   Precipitating Factors in Arthritis

The reader has probably noticed how frequently it has been necessary to say, "We do not know the exact cause." But we do know certain things that will precipitate arthritis. That is to say, certain things seem to start the disease or at times reactivate it after it has been quiescent. Although some of these have already been touched on, they are of sufficient importance for us to group them together in a single chapter and to repeat them, so that the patient may be on guard.

First of all is *fatigue*. Many times I have noticed in taking a patient's history that his arthritic attacks came after a period when he was fatigued, either physically, emotionally or both. Many times through this book I have pointed out that the patient must keep active. Keeping active is far different from working until the muscles and joints become exhausted and easy prey for the attack. I have seen cases of arthritis which seem to flare up in the springtime, because the patient after being indoors all winter decided to get outdoors and start a little spring gardening. The muscles were not used to it; and after a day's "relaxation"—trying to get the garden weeded so that it would look nice for the summer—the patient went to bed completely exhausted and the next day awakened to find that the arthritis had returned. Or patients who are working regularly and then find it necessary to spend unusual hours at work to get out fiscal reports, or meet writing deadlines; the work gets done but the arthritis comes back. Mental fatigue is just as important, and people who are under a heavy emotional strain are always in danger. This topic is discussed in more detail in chapter XI. But at this point the reader may be interested in a theory evolved by a Canadian physiologist, Dr. Hans Selye, known as the "Selye Adaptation Syndrome." Dr. Selye points out that when people (and animals, too, for that matter) are subjected to stress, certain reactions occur throughout the body which he calls the "alarm reaction." Now, in primitive man the stress which initiated this series of incidents was usually in the form of a physical challenge to him or to his home or food. The alarm reaction therefore mobilized all his bodily defenses for "fight or flight." But the stress which a man in the twentieth century faces is more likely to be a mixture of physical and emotional stimuli; a newspaper reporter jumping from one assignment to another and then filing his stories before the paper goes to press; a housewife with several children, doing the manifold chores of daily living; a busy contractor supervising several construction jobs and bidding on others. And the alarm reaction starts these twentieth-century mortals operating at their greatest efficiency, mentally alert and physically strong, as the Scouts say.

Then follows Dr. Selye's second phase, the stage of resistance. This is a continuing stage, when the body reactions do their work at an efficient pace. Now, compared with the resistance of the body, most stimuli last only a short time and the body is able to rest and be ready for new ones. But on occasions, stimuli may come one on top of the other without an adequate recovery period: the newspaper reporter is assigned to follow a political candidate's tour, listening to speeches all day and filing reports all night for several months; the housewife returns from the hospital where she has delivered her fifth baby to find one of the others sick with pneumonia and her husband gone with another woman; the contractor has a strike of workmen on one of his jobs, and is sued by an owner because of some defective plumbing found in another. In such cases the body may not be able to continue to respond to the increased and long-continued stimuli.

Then follows Dr. Selye's third and final phase, the stage of exhaustion. It is indeed, just this—when the body and mind are no longer able to keep up the pace—they become a ready prey for many illnesses, of which rheumatoid arthritis is one. Of course, everyone's capacity of resistance differs, some people will reach the stage of exhaustion much sooner than others. And in some people, the added stimuli may not be as dramatic as outlined. They may be just the nagging annoyances of an unpleasant job in unfavorable surroundings with an antagonistic boss, continued over many years. Finally it is too much—a break comes. Although it does not explain all the changes which take place, Dr. Selye's theory illustrates the necessity of adequate physical and emotional diversion throughout life.

The next important starting factor is *injury.* Many cases coast along well until an accident occurs and a joint is injured, following which there is a flare-up not only of that joint, but of the arthritis as a whole. Just why this should be is not entirely clear, but arthritics should take double precaution to protect themselves against falls and jolts and other things that will injure a joint already the seat of difficulty.

A generation ago *infection* was looked upon as probably the chief cause of many forms of arthritis, and particularly of rheumatoid arthritis. Today it is not listed so often. Yet it ranks high. Patients often get along well until they develop a sudden cold or an attack of virus, or kidney infection. Then they may have a return of the arthritis, which will last a long time. It behooves the arthritic to take all the sensible precautions he can to avoid precipitating his arthritis through the development of an infection.

Drafts and Exposure to Cold: Patients frequently feel that such factors have been responsible for their arthritis. Yet, scientific studies do not seem to bear this out. As will be explained in the next chapter, patients may feel worse under certain unfavorable climatic conditions, but it does not seem that the arthritis is brought about, or made worse, because of them.

Work: At times, a patient may blame his arthritis on conditions of employment. Rarely is this justified. Of course, if one's job causes serious physical or emotional strain, he should try to change it. But before radical steps are taken, a patient should make sure that the job, not himself, is at fault.

IX What Can Be Done About Arthritis?

To readers of this book who have arthritis, the question heading this chapter is the important one, probably the most important of their whole lives. Since, as we have seen, there are many types of arthritis and no one item is known to be the cause of all, it follows that there is no one single cure. Certainly the first lesson to be learned by the arthritic patient is that treatment in this group of diseases embodies diligent attention to all items of a well-rounded program and does not consist of the simple expedient of taking a certain number of pills or a series of "shots." The answer to "What can be done about arthritis?" is, "A great deal." This, however, has to be qualified with the statement that the exact nature and extent of what can be done varies with each individual. In discussing treatment of the rheumatic diseases, certain broad principles can be outlined, but the individual application can only be determined by the attending physician after a thorough investigation. Nowhere in the field of medicine is the general health of a patient so important as in the treatment of the rheumatic diseases. Since true specifics are rare and not universally effective, it is important that all those protective measures which nature has provided for the conquest of disease be maintained at their peak and fully used. In the treatment of arthritis, like so many things in life, an ounce of prevention is worth a pound of cure. So, the early institution of the measures, outlined below, will go a long way toward preventing serious difficulties as the years go by.

GENERAL MEASURES

Rest and Exercise: These two measures may at first be thought to oppose each other. On the contrary, they supplement each other. Adequate physical rest should be a main concern. First of all comes the question of sleep at night. This should include a minimum of eight hours, begun always before eleven p.m. Since the joints may themselves be painful at times and cause interruption to the sleep, whatever contributes to comfortable rest must be encouraged. Of prime importance is a comfortable mattress. It should be firm and not sag. A bedboard between an ordinary mattress and the springs may help, but if even this is not enough, a comfortable mattress of high quality is a sound investment. A single comfortable pillow should be available. It is essential that the bed be warm enough. An electric blanket usually permits comfortable sleep without too heavy covering.

In addition there should be an afternoon rest whenever possible. The best time is shortly after the noonday meal, and should be for an hour or an hour and a half. Although it is not necessary to sleep at this time, the patient should be lying down with all tight clothing, girdles, brassieres and shoes, removed.

An acutely inflamed joint may need even more rest than that obtained during the usual rest periods. A small splint, properly fashioned from metal, plaster, or one of the new plastics, may be applied to an inflamed wrist; or an arm may be held in a sling to protect an ailing shoulder. When the toes, ankles or knees are inflamed it may be necessary to stay in bed all day to avoid further irritation. Pillows and small sandbags may serve to hold the joints at rest and prevent strain.

The late Dr. Ralph Pemberton, who was the first American rheumatologist, once while addressing a group of doctors on this subject exclaimed, "Put your patients to bed for a week and watch the miracle nature will work." This, of course, was meant to be an exaggeration, but the principle is sound. Too often, patients feeling the necessity to "keep limbered up," fail to give the body the rest needed.

Suitable exercise, though, must be a part of the daily routine. This need not be strenuous and should never be overdone. It may be divided into two general categories; general body exercise and local exercise of a particular part. The former is to strengthen muscles throughout the entire body, to improve circulation through the organs as well as through the muscles; and to maintain good posture. All persons, whether arthritic or not, would be benefited by such a daily period of general body exercise. A list of such exercises will be found in Appendix B. In a healthy person the preferred time is in the morning on arising. Arthritic patients, however, may find it better to do these in the early afternoon, after a light lunch and before the afternoon rest period. Clothing should be loose and at a minimum. One must avoid fatigue in the exercise. Particularly is this true when resuming exercises after a long time without them. Excessive exercise at such times can cause damage through straining muscles. It is better to start slowly and gradually. The total amount in one day may vary, according to the patient's general feeling, the activity of his ailment at any particular time, and what else he does through the day. It should be between fifteen and thirty minutes.

Local exercise has for its purpose the maintenance or restoration of function in a specific area. This might be either the upper or the lower back, an arm, a leg, or a finger. In any joint that is the seat of acute inflammation or chronic deformity, exercise is needed. When a joint is acutely inflamed and kept splinted most of the day to avoid irritation and to aid nature in healing the inflamed tissue, it may become stiff from the formation of adhesions within. Therefore, at least once, and preferably twice a day, the splint must be removed, and the inflamed joint carried through as great a range of motion as possible. As the inflammatory reaction subsides, the joint should be exercised more and more. It is also possible to do much in this way toward restoring function in a joint that has become deformed from previous acute inflammatory attacks. The correction, however, may take months, or even years, and the therapeutic exercise regimen must be followed closely despite its monotony. A list of the exercises suitable for various parts of the body is given in Appendix B. It is not meant that all of the suggested exercises should be taken at one time; the attending physician can prescribe which particular ones are indicated and how long they are to be continued.

Diet: So much nonsense has been written about diet that I approach this topic a bit fearfully. Americans today are diet conscious. They have been told that millions in the United States are underfed, and that even those not underfed are likely to be undernourished. They have heard that special diets will cure high blood pressure, hardening of the arteries, ulcers, diabetes, gout, and nearly everything else. The many who are overweight keep looking for a special diet; one in which they can eat all they want and still reduce. So it is not strange that most arthritics should think there must be a diet which would cure arthritis; or if there is no diet to cure it, at least there should be foods to avoid and others to be taken in large quantities.

A successful lecturer on foods used to say, "We are what we eat." This to most people seems logical. The average person will say, "Of course we are." Yet it is true in only a small degree. You see, the body is an amazingly complex and marvelous organism. After you chew and swallow your food it is mixed in the stomach with certain digestive juices and then passed into the intestinal tract where it is mixed with other digestive juices. Your ham sandwich is not absorbed into your body as a chunk of bread and a piece of ham. The digestive juices have worked on it and the peristaltic motions of the stomach and intestines have chopped it up and changed it, so that it is absorbed into the blood stream as simple components—proteins, carbohydrates and fats. These are reconstructed in the body, primarily in the liver, and carried again by the blood stream to where they are needed, either to furnish energy or to build new tissues. It does not make much difference in the average healthy adult whether his protein building blocks come from a pig or cow, or for that matter, a horse or a goat. The important thing is that he gets his essential building blocks.

Now, I do not mean to say that diet is unimportant in the treatment of disease. Certainly a person with a stomach ulcer should avoid foods that irritate the ulcer. Diabetics have to avoid excessive intake of sugars, for they lack enough insulin to handle them. Later on, in the section on gout, we shall see why the gouty patient must avoid certain protein foods. But extensive tests seem to indicate that the arthritic patient has none of the physical abnormalities that require his limiting of certain foods. Nor will the taking of an excess of any particular food or vitamin alter his rheumatic state. Each of the vitamins has had a period of prominence when it was felt that that particular one, if taken in large doses, would aid the arthritic. Extensive trials and experiments now indicate that none of these has any significant curative effect. Indeed, the large doses of vitamin D, once recommended, may produce harmful changes in the body.

The average arthritic, like the non-arthritic, should have a well-rounded, nourishing diet, adequate in calories, but not excessive. Since there tends to be muscle loss in this disease, it is good to provide plenty of materials to form new muscles. These materials are best found in the protein foods. One readily available source of extra protein is in gelatin. Many arthritic patients find it helpful to take four to six envelopes of gelatin each day. This can be dissolved in water, in fruit juice, or in milk and drunk with meals or between meals. Included as Appendix A in this book are diets that meet these requirements.

Probably the greatest mistake of the average arthritic is overeating. This can become very troublesome, for the excess weight carried may damage the joints. Since the average person takes several thousand steps a day, one can realize how many thousands of pounds of damage can be done to ailing knees, ankles or lower spine by the constant pounding of extra weight. I wish I could put into this book a secret formula for reducing. There is none. One has only to read the myriad of special reducing diets appearing in the various women's magazines to appreciate how many overweight people there are and how hard it is to reduce. Each diet faddist tries to convince the patient that he can reduce without eating less. All such diets help the patient only to fool himself. There is no way to reduce without limiting the caloric intake, forcing the body to burn up the accumulated fat. Certain drugs on the market do help to the extent that they make the patient feel less hungry. Any of these, however, should be taken only on the prescription and advice of a physician.

No doctor can reduce a patient, but any doctor can show a patient how to reduce. It is quite true that one person may be able to eat more food without gaining weight than another can. Nevertheless, the original statement holds that everyone can reduce if he limits his diet. One has only to recall the wartime pictures of prisoners and civilian internees. All these people were thin and emaciated. Their diets had been limited and they lost weight.

A reducing diet need not be unpalatable. In the back of this book are diets of 2,400, 4,000, 1,400 and 1,000 calories. The first is a well-balanced diet for the person of average weight; the second is for the undernourished individual who is attempting to gain; and the other two are reducing diets. Several low-sodium diets (low-salt diets) are also listed. They should be used only under the direction of a physician.

The statement was previously made that no particular food will harm the person who has arthritis. But this statement, like any other about the human body, is subject to individual variation. Some arthritics do indeed note that their symptoms are adversely influenced by particular foods. I have several patients who say that whenever they eat concentrated sweets in the form of chocolate candy they find on the next day that their arthritis is worse. Others report difficulty after taking one or another of the citrus fruits, or tomato juice. On the other hand, I know a man who insists that the reason his arthritis has given him so few symptoms is that he has made it a point to drink a tall glass of orange juice every morning. Why then does one person seem to feel better and another worse when eating the same food? The answer is: personal idiosyncrasies or minor allergies. It is doubtless wise, when a patient has had a bad day, for him to think what food he has eaten during the last twenty-four hours. If he has had any unusual food, he should give himself a trial period later, both on and off this particular food to see if his system seems allergic to it. If so, then he should of course avoid it.

Also related to diet is the question of bowel regulation. Although a single daily bowel movement is the rule, it is by no means an essential or a necessity. Many normal persons have two or more movements a day; others only one every second or third day. True, patients who become severely constipated may note an increase in their arthritic symptoms. This constipation can usually be controlled by diet. A popular remedy for arthritis, which includes oranges, lemons, grapefruit and cream of tartar, owes its reputation to the simple fact that it is mildly laxative. It is much better to control bowels through diet, increasing the bulky foods and green vegetables and adding, if necessary, prune juice. If something more is needed, one of the bulk laxatives is preferable to other forms.

This seems a good place also to discuss alcohol and alcoholic beverages. The afternoon cocktail hour and the before-dinner cocktail have become so much a part of the life of many Americans that a person with arthritis may wonder if this will affect him. Now, alcohol physiologically dilates blood vessels, and temporarily improves the flow of blood into a joint. But there appears to be a secondary reaction to alcohol. Possibly the blood vessels undergo a secondary contraction. Whatever the actual physiology, most patients with arthritis find that they do not tolerate alcohol. An occasional drink may not cause trouble, but too many at one time, and daily drinks, should certainly be avoided. Patients with gout, as we shall see in a later chapter, must avoid alcohol entirely.

And what about smoking? To some people it seems almost as important as eating. Contrary to the action of alcohol, nicotine causes a contraction of blood vessels. Thus, when one smokes, the blood supply to his joints is restricted, but unlike alcohol, there is no secondary reaction, no improvement following the first effect. Hence, the action of nicotine is always to decrease circulation. It, too, should therefore be restricted to a minimum. A few cigarettes a day probably produce no difficulty, but those using a pack or more a day may be in for trouble.

Iron and Vitamins: A well rounded diet, as outlined in the appendix at the end of this book, will provide all the vitamins and minerals needed by the average patient. Under certain conditions, supplementary supplies are indicated. When that is true, they will be prescribed by the attending physician. The arbitrary use of vitamin pills "just to be on the safe side" is an expensive nuisance.

Climate: The effect of climate in altering rheumatic symptoms has long been legendary. Cold, damp, humid and rainy days are likely to make the patient more conscious of his symptoms, and warm, dry days usually bring a measure of relief. This kind of practical observation is now supported by scientific evidence. A special air conditioned apartment has been constructed within the Philadelphia General Hospital. Here, it is possible to alter climatic conditions—temperature, humidity, and ionization—without the patient's knowledge. Dr. Joseph Hollander and his group of research rheumatologists have observed patients under various "weather changes" for several months at a time. Their results indicate that many, but not all, patients experience increased symptoms during periods of falling temperature and falling barometric pressure. The exact reason for this is unknown, but it seems probable that it is related to the circulation, with the cold, damp weather causing a narrowing of the blood vessels supplying the muscles and the joints.

Still, there is no evidence that climatic factors significantly change the course of true arthritis, one way or the other, nor is there any scientific evidence to indicate that long-continued exposure to cold or dampness causes a flare-up from a dormant condition. However, because the patient feels his symptoms less, he will find that he does his best work in a warm, dry atmosphere.

The question often arises whether the patient should move to a different climate. Unfortunately, there are few places in the United States where the climate can be called ideal, and therefore desirable as a year-round residence for the rheumatic sufferer.

Both California and Florida have cold, damp seasons; the Midwest and the Arizona desert area both become cold in winter, and in the summer they are hot, making them uncomfortable for year-round living. On the whole, however, certain parts of Southern California, Arizona, New Mexico, Texas, and Florida do have enough warm, dry months to warrant being considered by the patient who shows persistent symptoms of generalized stiffness and aching. In deciding on a permanent move, other things besides the climate are of equal importance. It is of no benefit to a patient to move into a more equitable climate if he is not happy there. Separation from friends and relatives, or increased financial responsibilities, may produce an emotional upset far outweighing the ameliorating effect of the climate. It seems a safe statement that with all other factors equal, a move to a warmer, drier climate may be justified. The patient must realize, however, that this is not of itself going to cure his arthritis, although it may make him more comfortable and better able to live with it.

Spas and Mineral Waters: The virtue of healing waters has been extolled since ancient times. The practice of bathing in warm water or in warm springs to help relieve rheumatic pain dates to the time of the ancient Egyptians, and possibly earlier. "Watering places" were popular with the Greeks and Romans, and seeking benefit from baths was common throughout Europe in the Middle Ages. In more modern times both European and American spas have enjoyed financial success because of their popularity with rheumatic sufferers. That they helped temporarily to relieve symptoms, there can be no doubt; but that they are not curative is attested to by the number of people who return yearly for "the cure." The value of the spa is twofold. First of all is the local application of heat to the affected joint or muscle during the bath. In this respect it is similar to local applications of heat, either by the patient at his home or by the physician in the office. Second is the mental rest and relaxation induced by the general therapeutic regimen away from home and office worries. Drinking the water itself has no value whatsoever over and above the ordinary tap water found in any city. Some mineral waters are mildly laxative, so that their copious ingestion is equivalent to taking a mild dose of salts each day. Nothing in the mineral content of the water affects the arthritis. The advertising of mineral waters to be used in the home or office as a substitute for regular city water as a supposed aid in the treatment of arthritis is nonsense. Those taken in by this type of advertising are deluding themselves and wasting their money. In the Rheumatology Clinic at Georgetown University Hospital a series of arthritic cases were given a well-known mineral water while a similar number got ordinary tap water bottled to resemble the mineral water. At the end of the test no difference could be found between the two groups; those who had taken ordinary tap water felt as good and had progressed as well as those taking the mineral water.

Local Applications of Heat: Almost without exception, joints that are the seat of arthritis will be benefited by local applications of heat. This holds true whether the joint is inflamed temporarily or chronically, and even if there is deformity. The mode of application of heat differs. A joint acutely inflamed responds most satisfactorily to moist heat, best applied in the form of moist compresses. It is easy enough to wring a towel out of hot water and wrap the towel around the joint. The joints being treated should be at complete rest and not in an uncomfortable or strained position. Application of the compresses should be made two or three times a day for twenty or thirty minutes, never longer. They should be at a fairly constant temperature, neither too hot nor too cold. A patient often says that he has applied compresses "just as hot as I can stand them." This serves no useful purpose and may, indeed, be harmful. The heat should be just above body temperature; if checked with a thermometer, about one hundred to one hundred four degrees. Practical ways to keep the compresses at fairly even temperature are not difficult. Probably the easiest way is to place the warm, moist towel over the joint and then place on top of it an electric pad, set at the low heat. One must be sure that the pad so used is properly insulated to avoid short circuits when in contact with moisture. If such an electric pad is not available, a basin of warm water can be set beside the bed on an electric hot plate or grill, with the towel being wrung out of the water as needed. A convenient way to apply moist heat to the fingers is to exercise them in a basin of water. This is described in greater detail in Appendix B under "Exercises for the fingers." This same rule does not apply, however, to joints of the lower extremity, the ankle and toes. Here the patient would be sitting down and the forces of gravity would tend to make the feet swell after such applications of heat. To treat these joints one must be either sitting in a chair with his feet on a hassock, or else lying in bed so that the blood does not stagnate in the feet but circulates easily. Here compresses are most practical.

Chronically ailing joints are usually best treated by an infrared baking lamp. Fortunately the necessary apparatus is not costly. One can usually buy an infra-red bulb at a neighborhood drugstore at a modest price. This bulb is screwed into any light socket and is best used in a reading lamp or any gooseneck lamp that permits adjustment toward the joint being treated. It is best to start with the bulb two feet or so away. If it feels too warm, it can be moved back; if not warm enough, it is moved closer. A good deep heat is desired, not necessarily "as hot as you can stand." The heat output of lamps varies, and also a person's heat tolerance will vary from day to day; but in general, after a lamp has been used once the patient can readily determine just where it should be. Usually after two or three minutes' exposure it will be necessary to move the lamp farther away for the remainder of the treatment. If such simple precautions are observed it is not necessary to worry about a burn unless the patient falls asleep while taking his treatment. Unlike treatment with ultraviolet (where extreme caution must be used, and the exact time of exposure properly controlled), a patient will not burn from the infrared without knowing it. Each joint should be treated for about fifteen to twenty minutes twice a day; longer applications may produce congestion and do more harm than good. If a person does not have access to an infra-red bulb, other forms of heat can be used. Compresses can be made to do. An electric pad, or a hot-water bottle, or even a brick heated in an oven and suitably wrapped in towels, can answer the purpose.

An additional word about the infra-red bulb is probably in order. The term "infra-red" is used because this is the ray generated by such a bulb. It is also the ray put out by the heat pad and any other form of heat. Indeed, the heat ray is the infra-red ray. It is so called because it is just below (*infra*—below) the red ray in the visible spectrum. The infra-red ray is invisible; however, because in the popular conception an infra-red ray should be red, many heat bulbs are colored red by the manufacturer. These have no value over the clear bulb and put out exactly the same heat ray.

Another mode of application of heat that has gained popularity is warm paraffin. The paraffin block is melted in a double boiler and then allowed to cool to a point where a thin scum forms on top of the paraffin. Painful hands are dipped into the paraffin six to eight times until a thick coating of the hot wax covers the fingers and wrists. This is left on twenty to thirty minutes and then cracked off and replaced in the double boiler to be used over for the next application. This method of applying heat to the fingers gained favor some years ago, particularly in rural areas when large quantities of hot water were not easily available. It has no significant value over the warm water, and it is usually much more convenient for a person to exercise his hands in the basin of the bathroom.

Hormones: A discussion of hormones in this section of GENERAL MEASURES may surprise some people—for many believe their use to be quite specific in both the prevention and treatment of arthritis. Unfortunately, such is not the case. Now, since we have been concerned throughout this book with semantics, it would seem wise to clear up a point regarding the term we are using before going on with our discussion. To most laymen, the term "hormone" indicates a sex hormone—testosterone in men, estrogen in women. But from a medical standpoint, the sex hormones are only one of a large group of substances included in such a designation. Actually, a hormone is a product generated by any gland which empties its secretion directly into the blood stream and is therefore called an "endocrine gland." Thus, thyroxine from the thyroid gland, insulin from the pancreas, and cortisone from the adrenal are *all* hormones; while bile generated in the liver is not, for it passes into the intestinal tract and not directly into the blood. But popular usage makes "hormones" synonymous with "sex hormones," so we shall follow that routine in this discussion also.

Some years ago, physicians felt that the continued use of hormones might favor cancer formation. Happily, such fears have proved groundless. It appears now, that if properly regulated, ill effects from hormones are minimal provided there is no pre-existing cancer.

Unfortunately, the beneficial effects of hormones as treatment for any type of arthritis are not great. They have been recommended particularly in osteoarthritis, where it was hoped the aging process might be retarded, or even reversed. The idea is good but it just does not seem to work that way. However, hormones do have a definite place as supplementary treatment. They frequently help to overcome middle age depression in either sex—while their ability to eliminate the troublesome "hot flashes" during and following menopause has been one of the great boons to the "45 and up" woman.

Closely related to the matter of hormone therapy is the question of "the pill." Since patients with rheumatoid arthritis usually improve during pregnancy, it seemed logical to assume that the disease would undergo remission during "simulated pregnancy" as occurs when taking norethinol or other "progestational control" medications. Unfortunately, this has not been the case. Patients note little change in the course of their rheumatoid arthritis when taking these drugs.

Linaments and Ointments: Healing lotions and emollients have been applied to diseased and inflamed tissues since the dawn of man. In ancient civilizations, this was often done by the priest or witch doctor while he recited prayers or incantations. Yet, modern medicine appreciates that such local applications can be beneficial for they act as "counter-irritants." This means that when the skin is irritated there is a reflex dilatation of the underlying blood vessels. Thus, when linament is rubbed on the skin over an arthritic joint, there is an increased flow of blood into the joint itself. Various commercial preparations are available and unwarranted claims are, at times, made by the manufacturers. However, all are of approximately equal value. Ordinary oil of wintergreen which can be purchased quite cheaply at any drugstore is the equal of any. It is best to rub the oil lightly on a joint before retiring. The area is then wrapped in a wool or knit covering to retain the warmth generated. Ointments should never be applied prior to going out in the cold.

Protection of Joints Against Cold: This is probably a good place to mention that arthritics must take special care to protect their joints against undue cold and dampness. Warm clothing is a "must" during winter time. This includes wool gloves and knee warmers. In the same category, an electric blanket for use at night is an excellent investment.

DRUGS

The drugs which physicians prescribe for patients with arthritis can usually be divided into three categories. First are those which overcome the inflammatory reaction accompanying the arthritis; second, those which seem to have a specific action on the arthritis itself (used in rheumatoid arthritis); and finally, drugs prescribed to relieve pain.

In addition, one might also mention those drugs which are prescribed to improve the general condition of the patient, having only an indirect action on the arthritis (as hormones and vitamins previously listed).

ANTI-INFLAMMATORY DRUGS

Aspirin: Heading the list of anti-phlogistic drugs (those which help to relieve inflammation), is aspirin. It is the one medication generally recognized as being of benefit for virtually all sufferers of rheumatic diseases in nearly all stages of their illness. Aspirin is a salicylate, and its official name is acetyl salicylic acid. There are numerous other members of this salicylate family, all of benefit in arthritis and for similar reasons. These include sodium salicylate, amidopyrine, phenacetin and paraminobenzoic acid. Commercially, such drugs are available under a variety of names. The most common, besides plain aspirin, are Empirin, Anacin, Paba, Bufferin and Excedrin. Therapeutically they are all alike, each having the same effect on the patient's arthritis. Bufferin includes a medication designed to "buffer" or "neutralize" the stomach acid. In those patients who develop stomach upsets when taking plain aspirin, Bufferin may be a handy substitute. Various commercial preparations are also available in which the aspirin is coated so as to pass through the stomach and dissolve only in the intestines thus preventing stomach irritation. Paraminobenzoic acid (Paba), whose action is similar to salicylates, can be obtained in a sodium-free form and is, therefore, useful in patients who must be on a low-sodium diet. Empirin, Anacin, and Excedrin all contain a mild stimulant and, therefore, help to overcome the depression which some persons experience when taking salicylates. Acetaminophen, marketed under the trade name Tylenol, is a similar drug. It seems almost devoid of unpleasant side reactions but has not been available long enough to determine whether long continued use will be detrimental. Unfortunately, most patients do not find it as effective as aspirin.

The old prejudices against aspirin are slowly giving way in view of modern experiments. A generation ago, it was not uncommon for people to think aspirin "hurt the heart" or produced other unusual toxic effects. But, in general, salicylates are well tolerated and twelve tablets per day is a frequent dose. Some persons may experience ringing in the ears when taking this number and appropriate reduction is then indicated. The impaired hearing occasionally experienced disappears as the dose is reduced. Like all drugs, the prescription for aspirin must be coordinated by the physician.

Phenylbutazone (Butazolidin) and Oxyphenbutazone (Tandearil): These are also anti-inflammatory agents, somewhat more potent than aspirin. Phenylbutazone was developed in Switzerland as Irgapyrine, and first introduced in America in 1951. It has the property of relieving the pain and stiffness in many rheumatic diseases. Although primarily of benefit in gout and ankylosing spondylitis, it is sometimes effective in cases of rheumatoid arthritis, fibrositis, and osteoarthritis. There is a wide variation in the therapeutic response. Many persons taking only one tablet a day notice amazing relief of pain; others take up to four or five tablets a day without much benefit. Unfortunately, too, the administration of the drug is not always without side effects. These consist of skin rash, heart palpitation, fluid retention, stomach upset (at times even true ulcers) and depression of the blood forming mechanism. The actions and reactions of Tandearil are similar in all respects to those of Butazolidin. Some people seem to respond better to one than the other—which can be ascertained only by trial and error. A decision to use these drugs can be made only by the physician and patient together, with the expected benefits weighed against the possible dangers. By constant observation, adverse effects of such drugs can be kept to a minimum. However, no patient should agree to take them unless willing to assume part of the risk, for untold reactions, though rare, do occur even under close supervision.

Indomethacin (Indocin): This drug introduced in 1965 has proved to be another useful anti-inflammatory medication. Persons treated with this drug may respond dramatically, but many find no benefit whatsoever. Some develop side reactions (nausea, headache, dizziness, etc.), making it necessary to discontinue treatment. As is so often true in treating arthritis, trial and error is the only way Indocin's effectiveness can be determined.

Intravenous Nitrogen Mustard: This substance which has been used for some years in the treatment of leukemia has now been applied to rheumatoid arthritis. It is apparently helpful in temporarily relieving an acute inflammatory episode. It also seems useful in treating those patients who have gradually increased their steroid intake to dangerous levels, for after a course of nitrogen mustard, the steroid dosage can usually be sharply reduced. This drug, like Cytoxan discussed later under "specifics," will suppress the autoimmune mechanism if used over a long period of time. But since it is best given by intravenous injection, it is not suited for continuing therapy.

Artificial Fever Therapy: Since it has been observed that the inflammatory stages of rheumatoid arthritis may subside after a patient had had a fever, physicians have intentionally given patients medications which would bring about an elevation of temperature. These have included sterile milk injections into the buttocks, intravenous typhoid vaccine, and even malaria. When this is done, a temporary remission in the activity of the disease is usually noted. Although formerly quite commonly used, such measures are only rarely invoked at the present time.

Cortisone and ACTH: The most powerful of all the anti-phlogistic medications currently available are the cortisone derivatives and ACTH. Because of their importance, these hormones will be discussed in a separate chapter.

RHEUMATOID ARTHRITIS "SPECIFICS"

Most of the measures just outlined are general and suitable for use in all types of rheumatism. In addition to these, certain drugs used in treating rheumatoid arthritis are thought to have specific value in that disease, perhaps curative or arresting. New methods are constantly being developed and tried, but the ones listed below are the ones most commonly employed at the present time.

Gold: Probably the most useful drugs in treating rheumatoid arthritis are those compounds of gold referred to as "gold salts." They apparently have the property of acting on the underlying pathology of the disease. The use of gold for treating rheumatoid arthritis dates to about 1927, when a French physician, Dr. Jacques Forestier, first used it. At that time, physicians felt that many cases of rheumatoid arthritis might be tuberculous in origin and gold was being recommended as helpful in the treatment of pulmonary tuberculosis. It seemed logical to Dr. Forestier that gold might have a place in rheumatoid arthritis. Medical men now feel quite sure that rheumatoid arthritis has no particular relation to tuberculosis; and, furthermore, gold is no longer used in treating any form of tuberculosis. Nevertheless, the use of gold in many cases of rheumatoid arthritis has stood the test of time and is now an established method of treatment in all larger clinics throughout this country and abroad. The drug, however, is slow-acting and patients usually show no improvement for several weeks or months. Not all respond; the best results are usually obtained in early cases. Actually, it is not metallic gold which is used but a "salt" of gold, compounded to be readily absorbed and non-irritating. Preparations are available for injection either into a vein or a muscle. Unfortunately, gold is toxic and its use is always attended by possible danger. The most common complication of gold treatment is an itching skin rash. Damage may occur to the kidneys or to the bone marrow. Fortunately, medicines are available to combat such unpleasant side reactions. However, the fact that they may occur sometimes limits the usefulness of the drug, and even though precautions are taken, adverse reactions occasionally develop without warning and no patient should take gold unless he is aware of the facts.

Chloraquine Phosphate (Aralen) and Dihydroxychloraquine Sulfate (Plaquenil): Many cases of rheumatoid arthritis are benefited by these drugs, whose main usefulness is in treating malaria. Individual responses are quite varied but some persons show excellent improvement. Results may be delayed for many weeks after starting the drug. Like gold, chloraquine apparently acts directly on the underlying pathology of rheumatoid arthritis rather than on the inflammation which the pathology produces. Unfortunately, these drugs too, may have unpleasant side reactions. Some people experience gastric upsets. More serious, however, are certain eye complications which occur in a very small percentage of the patients taking the drug. Indeed, it seems wise for any person using either of these "anti-malarials" over an extended period of time to have regular eye checks by a competent ophthalmologist.

Cyclophosphamide (Cytoxan): In the chapter which discussed the causes of arthritis, it was mentioned that something seems to go wrong with the immunity mechanism in a person having rheumatoid arthritis (p. 36). So drugs which somehow suppress this "auto-immune" abnormality have been tried as therapeutic agents; and one that works is marketed commercially by the trade name Cytoxan. It has been used for some time in treating leukemia where it helps to reduce the excessive number of white cells in the blood (and hence, its name: *cyto*—cell; *toxan*—toxic). Although the dose used in treating rheumatoid arthritis is substantially less than that in leukemia, this tendency to reduce the white cells in the blood must be carefully observed whenever the medication is taken, and the drug stopped if the cell count drops too low.

Other side reactions may also be troublesome. At least half of those taking the drug lose their hair and still others develop cystitis with blood in the urine. Thus, it is not a medication to be taken lightly; but as is the case with other treatments for rheumatoid arthritis, some cases respond favorably to it when nothing else helps.

Antibiotics: As mentioned in the chapter on rheumatoid arthritis, some physicians believe infections may play a significant role in the cause of the disease. This has led to treatment with antibiotics. Although the results have not been spectacular, some patients apparently improve while taking these drugs. Lack of response generally could mean that no antidote has yet been developed for the infecting agent.

Nature's Methods of Treatment: Every patient suffering from rheumatoid arthritis knows that this disease has its "ups and downs." At times, the sufferer is able to put his finger on some happening which seems to have occurred just before the change in his condition is noted. He is apt to attribute the improvement or worsening of his condition to this episode, but this may be difficult to prove scientifically. Nevertheless, experience has demonstrated that remissions of rheumatoid arthritis frequently occur after a severe attack of jaundice, after an illness accompanied by high fever, and during pregnancy. It is believed that more than one natural phenomenon may be acting in such cases. Apparently various protective agents (such as the white blood corpuscles) are produced at an increased rate; then there seems to be an increased flow of blood through the various organs; and finally, various hormones which act on the inflamed tissues are produced in increased quantities.

PAIN RELIEVING DRUGS

In many cases the pain of arthritis can be severe, even devastating. All the drugs which have just been discussed will eventually help to relieve the pain by easing the arthritis—but there may be times when the patient feels he just cannot wait for this to take place and that he must have something to ease his pain immediately. Aspirin and its related compounds may be highly effectual. Other commercial synthetic compounds, such as Darvon and Zactirin, may also be used, but narcotics must be assiduously avoided. Even small doses of codeine can be the start of a dangerous habit leading to addiction.

ORTHOPEDIC REHABILITATION

In limited space one cannot go into all the details of orthopedic surgery and orthopedic rehabilitation applied to patients who have suffered severe damage to their joints from the arthritic process. Nevertheless, it should be said that today we have great hope for the restoration of many joints that have been severely damaged and formerly would have had to remain forever stiff and impaired. One of the best known surgical treatments is the insertion of a metal cap, or cup, into the hip. In this operation a severely damaged hip is opened, the surfaces smoothed over, and a metal cap inserted over the top of the end of the thigh bone. The joint is then closed and, after the wound has had time to heal, motion is started, slowly at first, but in gradually increasing degree. In many cases this proves quite satisfactory. But, sometimes the metal cup seems to become an irritant and the joint again stiffens. Because of this, experiments are being conducted with other operations. Artificial joints, or "prostheses" are being used to replace severely damaged ones. In such cases, the entire joint is removed and an artificial one inserted. When a hip joint is thus "replaced," a metal or plastic socket is bolted or glued into the pelvis and a metal ball replaces the top of the thigh bone. Metal and plastic finger joints may take the place of those made useless by arthritis. Tendons which have become frayed and torn, limiting the motion of fingers, can be stitched and repaired so as to restore function. Synovectomy—that is the removal of all or a part of the synovial membrane—is done to control a persistently swollen joint. Indeed, in some cases, synovectomy done early in the disease may prevent serious damage. Probably, in time, the various orthopedic operations will be refined and perfected and patients will be able to have their badly damaged joints repaired almost as easily as they have a gall bladder or an appendix removed. When that day comes, though, there may be little need of it, for we expect that the medical measures will bring the disease under control to the point where no joint will be so severely damaged.

X Cortisone and Like Drugs

Medical meetings at which doctors report to other doctors on their scientific investigations and discoveries are usually staid affairs. Papers are presented rather formally and the discussion and questions that follow are equally formal. But in 1949, when Dr. Philip Hench of the Mayo Clinic reported the results of his investigation of cortisone, the situation was different. First, at Atlantic City, where a group of young investigators formed the audience, and then later in the Waldorf-Astoria ballroom in New York where the members of an international congress on rheumatic disease were assembled, the usually dignified physicians, accustomed to giving a polite applause, not only applauded but stood up and cheered as though they had just seen Mickey Mantle hit one out of the park. The doctors realized that they were part of an historic occasion and that the events described would make medical history. Because cortisone is so important, and because every person taking it should have some knowledge of just how it acts, it seems sensible to tell of this in some detail.

First of all, cortisone is a naturally occurring and essential hormone. By this I mean that everyone's body generates some cortisone. If it did not, he could not live. A hormone, you will recall, is a product generated by one of the glands of the body and passed directly into the blood stream.

Now there are two small glands in the body, one on top of each kidney, called the adrenal glands. Years ago a hormone called adrenalin was isolated from these glands and most people know of it as a useful drug in combating shock. Scientists have known for years that this adrenal gland also generated other hormones, but the amount produced in a day, and the amount circulating in the body, is so small that their identification was for years impossible. Finally in the late 1930s, Dr. Edwin Calvin Kendall, a biochemist at the Mayo Clinic, succeeded in isolating five different compounds which he designated A, B, C, D, and E. One day as Dr. Kendall was discussing these compounds with some of his colleagues at the Mayo Clinic, Dr. Hench, who was in the group, was so impressed by what he heard that he made a note, "Try Kendall's compound E in rheumatoid arthritis." It was almost ten years before this note led to important results. First of all, the technical difficulties of producing the compound were enormous. It was impossible to get enough of the hormone from the glands of animals for experimental use. This meant that the chemical formula had to be determined and a way found to make the drug artificially. A full description of the tireless experiments and years of heartbreaking research that followed would fill volumes, but finally Dr. Kendall, working with chemists at the Merck Company, solved the problems and supplied Dr. Hench with small amounts of the new drug. And it worked! The first patient on whom it was tried was a man in the acute stage of rheumatoid arthritis who could barely walk or move his arms. Within three days after the hormone treatment was started he was up and about as though he had never had arthritis. Other patients responded immediately in a most favorable manner. This experience has now been duplicated in hundreds of thousands of cases. It can be said that almost without exception when cortisone is given in adequate doses to a patient with rheumatoid arthritis, the acute inflammatory symptoms of pain, swelling, redness, stiffness, can be eliminated.

But two other facts that Dr. Hench and his colleagues at the Mayo Clinic observed have also been amply confirmed by further investigations. The first is that cortisone is effective only so long as it is being administered. It does not cure; it only suppresses symptoms. The second is that when it is used for a long enough time, certain undesirable side reactions occur, some of them often serious. These include thinning of the skin with the appearance of spontaneous bruising, the retaining of fluid in the body, leading sometimes to dropsical conditions in the legs or abdomen, stomach irritation with even true ulcer formation, deposit of fat in various places, particularly around the face and neck, causing the so-called "moon face," increased facial hair in women, alterations in sexual desire, increased susceptibility to pulmonary tuberculosis, and weakening in the bones, especially in the back, which may even lead to collapse of some of the vertebrae. Furthermore, continuous administration of cortisone (or any similar steroid) may impair the function of the adrenal glands. It is as if they said, "If you are going to give this body cortisone, why should I? I will stop functioning." It may take the glands weeks or months to get back to normal if treatment has been carried on over a long period of time. For this reason, patients who have been taking cortisone and then suddenly stop, may suffer a relapse of their disease. And other symptoms of adrenal gland insufficiency may also appear—extreme weakness, fever, and in some cases, complete shock. At such times, the adrenal glands have difficulty generating extra supplies needed for emergency situations. A major operation is the most usual point in question. When this is performed under ordinary circumstances, the adrenal glands increase their secretion many fold; but the glands of a patient on steroid therapy are unable to do so. The patient must, therefore, be given supplementary cortisone intramuscularly. The surgeon will have ready additional supplies to be given if the patient's condition seems to require it.

Here then is a medication which in rheumatoid arthritis produces such dramatic relief of symptoms that it is properly called one of the miracle drugs, and yet it is also capable of producing side reactions just as serious as, or possibly even more so, than the arthritis itself. I frequently liken the use of the drug to the story of the boy who stopped the leak in the dike by holding his hand in the hole. The arthritis, while still there is not causing any damage. But as soon as the remedy is withdrawn, arthritis comes rushing back. Furthermore the constant pounding of the water against the hand and the natural fatigue of the work may injure the boy so that the hand has to be removed. So too, as the cortisone is used, side reactions may become severe enough to require its withdrawal. If the rent in the dike is small, materials may float down the river and produce a natural repair and when the hand is withdrawn, there is no further leak. Similarly, cortisone in certain early and mild cases of rheumatoid arthritis is permanently effective, but it cannot be relied on in most.

Since these things are true, how useful then is cortisone as applied to rheumatoid arthritis? First of all, cortisone is never given lightly or haphazardly, or without adequate control and supervision by a physician. Second, when a patient is taking the medication he must be acquainted with these possible side reactions and be on the lookout for them, to be able to advise the physician at their earliest signs. Finally, only the smallest possible dose must be used. This is perhaps the biggest single factor in controlling the side reactions. In fact the dose used now to control the arthritic symptoms is less than one-half of that at first recommended. True, control of the disease is not so complete with these smaller doses, but a logical compromise is sought; to give the patient enough relief from his acute symptoms for him to continue his activities, but without attempting to eradicate the symptoms entirely. Readers of this book who do not suffer from a severe form of rheumatoid arthritis might say, "I would never take that drug." But in some cases rheumatoid arthritis can be so devastating that one is glad to risk heroic treatment.

Since the original discovery of cortisone there has been a constant search for other hormones which would relieve the arthritis, but would not produce the undesirable side reactions. The first of these discovered was hydrocortisone, also a hormone occurring naturally in the adrenal gland. Although slightly more powerful than cortisone, its adverse reactions are just as severe. And since its cost of production is higher than that of cortisone, its worth is not much greater than cortisone itself. Of the many thousands of hormones which have been developed and tried since these two, only a few others have been found to be of practical value. Two of these were discovered by chemists at the Schering Corporation laboratories. They named their compounds Meticorten and Meticortelone and these are still the most popular terms for these drugs, although the official names are Prednisone and Prednisolone respectively. Other companies now making the same drugs have other names but they are the same product. These drugs are four to five times as powerful as their predecessors and many of the unfavorable side reactions are less. Unfortunately, the side reactions even with these have not been completely eliminated and the same precautions must apply. So the search continues; at present, there are more than ten such compounds available. Because of their chemical nature they are spoken of as "steroids" and it is, therefore, proper to say that more than ten different steroids are now available for the treatment of rheumatoid arthritis. Each possesses subtle differences from the others, having advantages and disadvantages. Unfortunately, the perfect steroid hormone has not been found. Which one is best in any particular case is up to the individual physician who is prescribing for that case.

ACTH (corticotropin), too, is of great use. The letters ACTH stand for "adrenal cortex trophic hormone," meaning that it is a hormone that will stimulate the adrenal cortex to produce its own cortisone. ACTH is secreted by that master gland-regulator, the pituitary gland, hidden deep in the skull below the main lobes of the brain. This gland is a truly remarkable one, for it generates secretions that seem to control all the other glands. It was only a short time after Dr. Hench discovered cortisone that one of his colleagues, Dr. Charles Slocumb, obtained some ACTH from the Armour Laboratories and proved that this, too, will control rheumatoid arthritis by making the patient generate in his own body more cortisone than normally. In other words, whether a person takes cortisone that has been manufactured artificially, or takes ACTH and stimulates his own adrenal gland to produce excessive cortisone, the final result on the rheumatoid arthritis is the same. However, side reactions are also the same, and since ACTH must be given by repeated injections through the day, this method has its drawbacks.

In addition to their value when given by mouth to patients

with rheumatoid arthritis, both hydrocortisone and prednisolone are of value when injected directly into joints. Not only joints swollen and painful from rheumatoid arthritis will respond, but also those stiff and sore from osteoarthritis. Fortunately, also, the side reactions mentioned do not occur when the drug is thus given directly into the joint. Consequently, if only a few joints are involved, intraarticular injections may control the condition. Because cortisone may lower resistance, there is always the possibility that repeated injections may lead to infection and adequate precautions must be taken.

So many variations occur that nearly everything said in this chapter about dosage and administration is subject to modification. One patient may be controlled on 5 or 7.5 mgm of prednisone while another may require more. Some patients develop side reactions after taking the drug only a few days—others can continue for months with minimal difficulty. It is for this reason that the patient and physician must work in close cooperation and realize that even though a physician may have treated thousands of cases, each new one presents a new aspect.

Because these drugs are now widely used, and discovery of each new advance is profitable not only to the patient, but to the drug manufacturer, every pharmaceutical company is vitally interested in providing a new and better drug for the patient. This is most encouraging and there is reason to believe that drugs will finally be developed having strong anti-arthritic value and only minor side effects.

XI Mental and Emotional Factors in Rheumatic Diseases

Perhaps it would be well to introduce the discussion of this topic by a case report.

"Are you trying to tell me, Doctor, that I am just imagining all the pain because my husband and I don't get along?"

She was a young-looking woman of forty, who had first consulted me a week before, because of pains in her hands and arms.

On her previous visit, I inquired thoroughly into her medical history and had her return after two days for a complete physical examination, laboratory studies and x-rays. These had all shown only the mild, early osteoarthritic changes to be expected at her age. Her symptoms were more severe than the findings could possibly explain, and I then suspected some other cause—perhaps an emotional upset. She was now back in my office to receive the reports and recommendations.

I had reviewed the x-rays with her, pointing out the small changes, and told her that the rest of my examination had shown her to be in excellent health. Although she expressed gratitude for being found in good health, she still seemed disappointed, for she had assured me that she had "a bad case of arthritis." I then asked her if she did not think her husband, too, would be gratified to learn that her arthritis was less severe than she had feared. She sat up a little straighter, shrugged, looked out of the window and replied, "He says there's nothing wrong with me anyhow."

That opened the door to a detailed discussion of her marital relationship. On her first visit she had avoided details of her home life, simply saying that she lived at home with her two children and that she and her husband got along "quite well, about average, I guess, for people married fifteen years." The pattern she then described was a familiar one. Her husband held a fairly responsible job in a government agency in Washington, head of a division, with a staff of workers, both men and women under him. He often had to work overtime, particularly when budget estimates or yearly reports were being prepared. He had entered government service immediately after college and had advanced himself because of his ability and a willingness to do the overtime work without complaint. His salary was enough to meet the family needs. He spent about two nights at the office each week; another evening he usually devoted to a civic club, and still another as a member of a bowling team. She said he spent Saturday and Sunday mornings sleeping, Saturday afternoons watching television, and Sunday afternoon at golf. When he did have an evening at home he was usually "too tired to do anything but read the paper and go to bed." No, she replied to a specific question, she did not think he was interested in any other woman, and besides "it wouldn't make too much difference if he were." She had always felt that she and her husband were sexually compatible, although he had never been too eager even when they were first married. In recent years his desire had apparently declined and now they frequently went two to four weeks without love-making. When they did make love, it seemed satisfactory, though her husband never showed much enthusiasm.

Resentment of her husband's attitude seemed evident, and yet when I intimated that there might be a connection between her feeling of rejection at home and those painful hands, she challenged me with the question I have quoted.

"No," I told her, "I'm not at all saying that you're imagining the pain. Of course it's there, and it is a distressing pain. What I am saying is that the arthritis alone would not cause that pain.

"Let's see if I can make this a little clearer. We'll forget arthritis for a minute and talk about something entirely different. Take blushing. When you blush, the small blood vessels, the capillaries, in your face open and the blood cells come out of the capillaries into the cheeks, making the cheeks red. The blood is then absorbed back into the capillaries and when you stop blushing your face shows its normal color. Now what was it that made you blush? Maybe you had been talking about something to a friend, perhaps a small bit of gossip and all of a sudden you looked up and the person you were talking about was there and had overheard. You were embarrassed, and so you blushed. Now you didn't want to blush. There wasn't any physical stimulation of the blood vessels in your face. Just certain wheels went around, as you might say, up in your brain and then the blood vessels in your face opened up.

"Let's have another illustration. Did you ever have a lump in your throat? Were you ever at a meeting, maybe at the PTA, when you were called on to speak and didn't know what to say? All of a sudden you got a lump in your throat. You couldn't talk because there was a feeling of constriction in your throat. You didn't imagine that constriction; it was there. The muscles in your throat contracted and held you speechless. But here again nothing touched those muscles; there wasn't any physical stimulus.

"Another illustration is tears. Probably you've been to a play or a movie when a scene made you cry. You didn't stimulate your tear glands by touching them. It was just that from certain emotions aroused inside your brain your tear glands begin to secrete.

"So you see, we have blood vessels altering their characteristics, muscles contracting, and glands stimulating, and all on a purely emotional basis. Now, these illustrations are all momentary ones. But if the stimulus were continued over a long period of time, certain permanent changes would occur in the blood vessels or muscles which would permanently alter their characteristics.

"And when I say your arthritis can be affected by your emotions I am not saying that you just imagine your arthritis is worse; it really gets worse. When you are under emotional strain the blood vessels alter, the muscles alter, the glands which control other secretions and carry various hormones to your joints alter. All this adversely affects your arthritis."

This is what is meant by "psychosomatic" conditions. *Psycho* means mind and *soma,* body; so this is a condition in which the body is influenced by the mind.

I could give many illustrations to point out these facts. There was a woman who lost two sons within a month of each other toward the end of the war. All of a sudden her end finger joints became swollen and red and tender, primarily from psychosomatic stimuli. Finally, the condition quieted down. Two years later the boys were brought home for reburial and—presto!—all over again, her hands got stiff. She was not imagining the swellings in her hands. She could see them and I could see them, but the psychic influence she lived through twice, when the sons were killed, and then reburied, caused this severe return of her arthritis.

Another woman was injured in a street-car accident. She developed arthritis of her end finger joints, within a few months. The fingers themselves had not been injured in the accident; but the emotional shock she had gone through manifested itself in the arthritis.

I think of a woman who nursed a sick mother through a severe illness. The mother had cancer and for the last year of her life was bedridden. Her only daughter had to take care of her. There wasn't enough money to hire a nurse or even a full-time companion, so the daughter got up in the morning, took care of mother, by bathing her, prepared her breakfast, set her lunch alongside her, and then went off to the office. In the evening she came home, tidied her mother up again, served her supper, and got her ready for bed. In the last few months it was even necessary for her to run home from the office at noontime. For over a year this woman lived under a severe physical strain, but the emotional strain was just as great. She was the only child and all her life she and her mother had been close. As she saw her mother go downhill and finally die, it brought on a severe emotional disturbance. Within a month after the mother's death she developed a severe case of rheumatoid arthritis that was difficult to treat.

Many people's ailing joints may indeed be related to deep-seated psychiatric difficulties. In such cases the attending physician may need help from a psychiatrist before the problem can be resolved. But this is more apt to be true in so-called psychogenic rheumatism, where no true arthritis exists but the patient "fixes" on his joints and develops complaints due, not to arthritis, but to his need to escape from situations that his emotional state will not permit him to face. The underlying disturbance may be quite obscure and be found only after intensive psychiatric investigation.

Other cases of psychogenic rheumatism are more obvious. These are usually the people of age forty and over who develop mild muscular aches and pains incident to their age, and who immediately are sure they are about to come down with a severe case of arthritis. They are usually the chronic emotional people who have been worriers all their lives. Often they have had a relative, possibly a father or a mother or an uncle, or other associate, who has had a severe arthritis. Now, with each new ache or pain, they are sure that they, too, are about to have a crippling disease. Emotionally unstable to start with, they are likely to develop symptoms from the slightest causes. In this same group are often found the people who cannot accept the idea of growing old. As the years pass and their physical energies slow down, they find all sorts of excuses and almost seem to prefer some kind of physical illness rather than accept the fact that the years inevitably take their toll.

In view of what has been said, a person with arthritis may well wonder just how important to him is the question of mental and emotional upset. Is it a small factor? Is it a moderate one? Or is it the sole cause? Different physicians give different answers. But all agree that emotions play a large part. I have frequently told patients that, although I am not yet convinced that emotions are the main cause of arthritis, I am sure that emotions play a big part in determining the course of the arthritis once it develops. By this I mean that if a person has arthritis, his feeling about the disease and his environment govern whether he will be able to handle the disease well, and handle himself well, or end up as a chronic invalid. I often think of a woman who consulted me some years ago. She had had arthritis for thirty years and was in her mid-fifties. She had moderate deformity of her hands, as well as the knees and feet. She walked with a slight shuffle and used her hands a bit clumsily, but on the whole she got around and did her work well. In our original consultation I asked her, "Just how much work can you do?" "Everything," she replied. "Let me tell you a story, Doctor. A friend of mine who used to live in the same city I did—in fact only a block away from me—developed arthritis the same year I did. There was just one difference. She had lots of money and I didn't. As soon as she developed arthritis she began to feel sorry for herself. She spent the next ten years of her life, and much of her husband's money, going from doctor to doctor trying to find a sure cure. In addition, she had nurses to wait on her and did almost nothing herself. In fact, she was carried at all times from her home, even to her back yard. It wasn't possible for me to do that, for I had to be out working every day, so I went to the doctor and told him, 'With your help and God's we're going to beat this.' I can't say we've beaten it entirely, but I've lost very few days from work, because I've kept after it and kept on my feet. I've had to; she didn't."

I have seen that woman's attitude—and her friend's—repeated over and over. Indeed, both are well known to every physician who treats much arthritis. When a patient comes into my office and says, "Doc, I'm going to beat this blankety-blank thing," I always say, "I'm sure you will." But when a person comes in with a long face and cheerfully says, "Doctor, do you think I'm going to end up in a wheelchair?" I usually look the patient in the eye and say, "That depends on you; you can give in to it, but you can also keep walking, if you really want to."

True, all this is easier said than done. There are times when arthritis is painful and when a person really wants to stay in bed and just sit and rest, but the old revival hymn, "Yield Not to Temptation," has in it an appropriate line. It says, "Each victory will help you some other to win." I don't mean that a person must keep exercising and keep on his feet until he drops from exhaustion. Indeed, elsewhere I have cautioned against fatigue. But

I most certainly mean that one cannot fall into the habit of sitting in the chair and calling for someone else to do the work.

So much for the sticktoitiveness part. This still hasn't solved the problem of unpleasant family relationships and arthritis. This comes under the heading of "adjustment," a word so much used today. A book of this type cannot possibly tell each person how to solve his or her personal problems, but these problems must be solved, with psychiatric help if necessary. For so long as they go unresolved, the emotional seeds for arthritis (and indeed for many other diseases, including high blood pressure, ulcers and heart disease) may be sown.

Many of the troubles seem to stem from selfishness, sometimes on the part of the patient, sometimes on the part of another member of his family, a husband, a wife, an in-law, a child. These problems could be solved perhaps by one member of the family showing more consideration for the other. A patient will not ordinarily accept the idea that the fault is his own. He sees only the fault of the other members of the family and when an attempt is made to point out that some of the fault rests with himself, the physician is told that he just does not know the situation. Sometimes it is true that the patient has made every effort to heal a breach in family relationships, but has been unable to do so. If a person must then go on living in such an environment, he must make up his mind that he can adapt himself to it. For his own emotional and physical well-being he must learn to adjust. That can mean making life so full that there is no time to feel sorry for oneself. It should not be necessary to tell a person how to keep his life full, and yet it seems that it often is. I am continually amazed at how blind people are to opportunities for service which abound in every neighborhood. Every hospital is crying for volunteer workers to help out in the crowded wards among the sick and severely disabled, or to assist as volunteer workers in the clinic. I know a woman who forgot her own arthritis and has been greatly improved just by helping out in the arthritis clinic in a large hospital. She has had to spend so much time helping others to solve their problems that she doesn't seem to have time to think of her own.

If one does not like hospital work, there are many other avenues of social service open. Volunteer workers are needed among the various health agencies. Not only the Arthritis Foundation, but the Heart, Polio, Cancer and Muscular Dystrophy foundations and united community services can use people who have the time and talent to help in their complex programs.

Nearly everyone has heard of Alcoholics Anonymous. That organization will not attempt to help a man who is a chronic alcoholic unless that man first of all wants to be helped, and second, unless he admits that it is not possible for him to help himself on his own strength alone, but must appeal to a higher force. The formula works. Thousands of people in our country today, who but for the help of Alcoholics Anonymous would be drunkards, are now living useful lives. I am not suggesting that we form a "Rheumatics Anonymous." What I am pointing out is that it is often necessary to admit that one has a problem and then say, "With God's help, I will bear it." Fortunately, today most clergymen, Protestant, Catholic, or Jewish, well know the great need for spiritual guidance in the everyday life of their parishioners. All are willing to give help, even to those who have not been too faithful. Spiritual guidance can be more important than medical guidance, but until the patient is willing to do his part both doctor and clergyman are powerless. Patients often delude themselves. They tell me, "Oh, Doctor, I pray so hard that I can get well," and yet they are not willing to do their own part. They do not admit it, but they are enjoying their own misery because it is the one thing that helps to center attention on themselves.

This is not meant to be a universal indictment of all arthritics, for many are hard-working, stable, God-fearing people. But it is meant to stimulate every chronic rheumatic sufferer to examine his life and determine if emotional problems are retarding his recovery.

XII   Laboratory Procedures

In this day of scientific study and progress, when even a young child may know the theory behind the splitting of the atom and take for granted the measurements of airplane speed and television wave-lengths, both physicians and laymen are likely to rely heavily on laboratory tests in diagnosing and treating any disease. In the rheumatic diseases, however, laboratory tests play a far less important part than in many others. Although certain tests are necessary to follow the clinical course of the disease, nevertheless the patient's symptoms and the appearance of his joints are a better index than the tests which we now have available. Since the patient with arthritis will probably find his physician checking various laboratory procedures, it may be wise for him to know what the doctor is doing and what he is looking for.

The Blood Count: As most persons now know, blood is made up of two main parts. First, there is the thin, straw-colored fluid called serum, and second, the blood cells which float in the serum. The pumping action of the heart keeps these blood cells well mixed so that there is a uniform distribution. Now the cells are of two main types, red cells, called erythrocytes (*erythro*—red; *cyte*—cell) and white cells, called leukocytes (*leuko*—white). Actually the red cells are a bluish-red color and since they are far more numerous than the white cells, it is they that give blood its color. The number of each type of cell within the serum is important, but since they are so numerous, it is necessary to dilute the blood before they can be counted. Almost everyone has seen a laboratory technician prick a person's finger with a small blade and then draw up a fraction of a drop of blood into a glass pipette. If this procedure is observed carefully, it will be noted that the technician draws the blood into the stem of the pipette and then dips the pipette into a clear fluid and draws a large quantity of this into the pipette. The pipette is then shaken well to distribute the cells uniformly and a drop of this diluted blood is placed in a special counting chamber under a microscope. The technician then counts the number of cells in a given area and by making the necessary corrections for the dilution can then estimate the actual number of cells. Since there are two types of cells to be counted, it is necessary to draw up two types of diluting fluid into two separate pipettes. One diluting fluid dissolves the white cells, but leaves the red cells intact so that they can be counted, while the other dissolves the red cells, keeping the white cells intact. The normal person has between four and five million red cells per cubic millimeter of blood and between five and nine thousand white cells in the same amount. When one considers that there are approximately thirty thousand cubic millimeters to each ounce, and that there are approximately seven quarts of blood in the body, it can be seen how many million separate cells are contained in the blood. Truly, the human body is a marvelous machine. Although the red cells are of fairly uniform size, this is not always true and it is therefore important to know the total volume which the red cells occupy in relation to the blood. This is not hard to determine. A specimen of the blood is collected in such a way as to make sure it remains fluid and does not clot. It is then placed in a centrifuge for a measured time. When the tube containing the blood is removed, it will be found that the blood cells have packed at the bottom of the tube. The proportion of the total space which the red cells occupy is spoken of as "volume percent of red cells" or "the hematocrit." In the average healthy person this figure will approximate 44, meaning the 44% of his blood volume is made up of red blood cells.

Now the main purpose of the red cells is to carry the iron-bearing compound, hemoglobin, around the body. The amount of hemoglobin which each cell contains may be altered. It is possible to estimate the total hemoglobin present in any given quantity of blood by chemical means which dissolve the red cell membrane, leaving the hemoglobin to combine with the particular chemical used. This produces certain color changes which can be compared with the standard in a colorimeter and thus the actual amount of hemoglobin measured. It is possible to determine not only the total red cell count, but also the total hemoglobin content and so tell whether there are too many or too few red cells, and whether each cell contains sufficient hemoglobin. A deficiency in the total number of red cells present, an abnormal lowering of the hematocrit, or a deficiency in the amount of hemoglobin present is spoken of as "anemia." Actually this word means "without blood" (*an*—without; *haemia*—blood), but no one, of course, is actually without blood, or he would also be without life. The term is relative.

Like all tissues in the body, blood is constantly being changed. That is to say, the bone marrow is constantly forming new cells and various tissues, particularly the spleen are destroying the old ones. In the patient with rheumatoid arthritis, both of these processes may, at times, be altered. His tissues may destroy cells more rapidly than is customary and his bone marrow may not form cells as efficiently. Consequently, a rather troublesome anemia frequently occurs. Furthermore, this may be quite resistant to the usual measures of iron and vitamins taken by mouth or injection. Only transfusions may correct the anemia and even these only temporarily.

The normal white cell count, while usually varying between five and nine thousand, may show even greater extremes. The chief purpose of the white cells seems to be to resist infection and consequently when an infection is present the body usually increases the number of white cells circulating in the blood to attempt to combat it. When rheumatoid arthritis is in an acute fulminating stage, the white cell count usually goes up. This is one of the things that has led doctors to suspect an infection as the cause, yet other factors have not always borne out this theory. Since the white cells seem to be particularly vulnerable to certain medications (as for instance gold and Butazolidin) it is necessary to keep a check on them while these and other drugs are being administered. If the white cells begin to fall, it is usually an indication to modify the treatment.

Just to complicate matters there are various types of white cells with such interesting names as polymorphonuclear leukocytes, lymphocytes, monocytes and eosinophiles. Determining their separate percentages in the total white cell count is known as "the differential count." The physician will want to know these totals, but they are rarely of importance to the patient.

Urinalysis: Kidney damage is usually not a part of arthritis, except in systemic lupus erythematosus and progressive systemic sclerosis (scleroderma). However, a patient with arthritis may also be suffering from other ailments which will cause damage to the kidney and thereby impede his progress or recovery. For this reason physicians are always interested in a study of the urine, both by chemical and microscopic procedures. Here, too, certain medicines may damage the kidney, necessitating frequent checks of the urine while they are taken.

Blood Chemistry: The yellow liquid blood serum contains a number of chemicals which the body uses. Not many of them are significantly altered in arthritis. Uric acid, which is so important in gout, will be discussed later. The blood proteins, on the other hand, may show interesting variations. The two chief proteins in the blood are albumin and globulin. Although both of these can be broken down into further components, a detailed discussion of these is not practical in this book. Usually there is about three times as much albumin as there is globulin in the blood, yet in cases of active rheumatoid arthritis this ratio is frequently reversed. The full significance of this is not yet clear, but the finding occurs often enough to indicate some basic change. We do know that a certain portion of the globulin—the "gamma globulin"—carries most of those protective mechanisms of the blood called "immune factors." Every mother with young children will recall an epidemic when the authorities recommended that the children, who have not had that particular disease, be given gamma globulin as a protective measure. So the rise in globulin noted in rheumatoid arthritis seems to indicate that the body is trying to form its own protection against the disease. This view is further supported by the fact that the gamma globulin itself has many subdivisions—and these subdivisions may vary in different diseases. Unfortunately, no specific immune globulin now exists which can be given to the patient to aid in the treatment.

In addition to the factors mentioned, physicians, studying patients with arthritis, will frequently wish to check other chemical constitutents in the blood such as sugar, urea, cholesterol or iodine content in order to determine the patient's general condition, and to outline the proper treatment.

Blood Sedimentation Rate: This is one blood test which most sufferers from rheumatoid arthritis have heard discussed, yet very few seem to understand. Most persons seem to have the idea that it is a measure of some unusual sediment that forms in the blood. Actually such is not the case at all; it is rather a measure of the speed with which the cells will settle out from the liquid when the blood is left to stand. As mentioned previously in this chapter under a discussion of the blood count, the blood itself is made up of two main elements, the liquid serum and the solid cells which constantly float in the serum. Now if blood be drawn from any person, sick or well, mixed with something to keep it from clotting and then placed in a glass tumbler and set aside overnight, it will be noted in the morning that the blood has separated into two layers. At the top is the thin, yellow liquid serum and below is the thick solid blue-red cells packed together. If the container in which the blood is held is now shaken it can be mixed to its former consistency. If again set aside, it will again separate into the two layers. The speed with which this settling-out process takes place has been found to be significant. In many diseases, and particularly in rheumatoid arthritis, the settling process takes place more rapidly than occurs in the normal blood. To check this clinically a uniform test has been devised. A measured amount of blood is mixed with a measured amount of anticoagulant and then placed in a standard tube. The tube is filled to the top where there is a line marked zero; down the tube are other markings, one, two, three, four, five, etc., one millimeter apart. After the tube has been filled it is placed in a rack for one hour and at the end of that time the point where the separation of the serum and the blood cells occurs is noted. This point is called the sedimentation rate (a more descriptive term would be the "settling point"). Since it is the red cells which are primarily concerned in this settling, it is often spoken of as the erythrocyte sedimentation rate, which is abbreviated ESR. Most persons in good health will have a sedimentation rate of 15 or less. In rheumatoid arthritis, the higher the sedimentation rate, the more active the disease is apt to be. The test, however, is not specific nor is it infallible. Usually when a person has had an active rheumatoid arthritis with a high sedimentation rate, the rate will fall as he improves clinically. However, a certain number of persons will retain a high rate regardless of improvement. Also, as the years go by many older people will show a high sedimentation rate without any apparent evidence of disease.

Test for "Rheumatoid Factor": When discussing the blood chemistry, we mentioned that the globulin fraction of the blood protein contains various protective substances known as "immune bodies." This name has been applied since they develop in the blood after a disease has started and help a patient combat that disease. In some diseases (scarlet fever, typhoid fever), they protect against future attacks. In many cases of rheumatoid arthritis, the patient's body develops a substance in the globulin fraction which is apparently an immune body and which has been termed "rheumatoid factor." As part of its protective mechanism, this factor has the peculiar ability to cause certain small particles of material to clump together, a process which is known as "agglutination." The red blood cells taken from a sheep—or microscopic latex particles—or bentonite clay particles, if suspended in suitable material, will be "agglutinated" when serum from patients with rheumatoid arthritis is added to the suspension. A test based on this finding is helpful in diagnosing rheumatoid arthritis. Although not 100% accurate, it is often of great help in questionable cases.

X-rays: The x-ray is probably the most useful laboratory test we have for following the various forms of rheumatic diseases, but even x-rays have their limitations. This is because an x-ray is quite different from a photograph. If you ever had your chest x-rayed you will recall that you stood facing the metal cassette which held the film, with the x-ray tube behind you. So, too, when a hand or other joint is being x-rayed, the film is placed on one side and the x-ray tube on the other. Now as the x-ray beam passes through the part being photographed, the rays will be stopped by dense bone, but will pass through skin, blood vessels and cartilage; the x-ray negative will show gray and white tones for bone and darker tones for the softer tissues. You may recall that in our discussion of the development of the various forms of arthritis, it was mentioned that all forms usually start rather slowly, and that the first changes occur in the synovial lining in rheumatoid arthritis and in the cartilage in osteoarthritis. Since both these structures are less dense than bone, rather extensve changes can be taking place in these membranes without being recorded on the x-ray. As times goes on, however, and the cartilage is destroyed, either in rheumatoid arthritis or osteoarthritis, the bones come closer together and this "narrowing of the cartilage space" can be seen on the x-ray. Eventually rather prominent changes may take place in the bone itself. It may lose its calcium and show on the x-ray as osteoporosis (*osteo*—bone; *porosis*—porous), or it may be eroded away in cystic-like areas, or the ends of the bones may be fused (ankylosis). Although the changes in the x-ray may not be diagnostic for a particular form of arthritis, nevertheless they do help considerably in following the progress of a case, for they show advancing changes as the disease progresses.

L. E. Preparation: As mentioned earlier in this manual, the disease known as systemic lupus erythematosus has recently attracted considerable attention. One of the factors which gave great impetus to this investigation was the discovery that in this disease certain changes take place in some of the white blood corpuscles. The test is somewhat complicated, for unfortunately the change which is taking place in the white cell cannot be observed by simply looking at the white cells under the microscope.

Instead the blood has to be prepared in a special manner. Furthermore, the change may not take place in a very large percentage of the white cells. Consequently, after the blood has been carefully prepared a rather diligent search must be conducted on the microscope slide to find the cell. It may even be necessary to repeat this several times. Although tedious and time-consuming, and therefore somewhat expensive, the identification can be most useful, for it may help to clarify a complex problem. Other tests for systemic lupus utilize the "agglutination reaction" described previously for rheumatoid arthritis with certain appropriate modifications made to identify a "lupus factor."

PART TWO

XIII   Introduction to Gout

Gout is an ancient and an honorable disease. Its painful attacks have plagued man since antiquity and its strange course has intrigued physicians ever since they began seriously to study the nature of diseases. It was recognized by Hippocrates of ancient Greece, whose "Hippocratic Oath" written more than four hundred years before the birth of Christ, still stands as the ideal of medical ethics. Even before that, however, Egyptian physicians were prescribing for the disease. Hieron of Syracuse in the fifth century B.C., apparently recognized it, for he commented on the association of bladder stones and joint disease, something that occurs in gout, but not in other rheumatic conditions. The chalky bodily deposits of gout, called tophi, were described by the Roman physician, Galen, who lived in the second century A.D. In this same period, Aretaeus of Cappadocia noted its preponderance in men and also mentioned the fact that the great toe is frequently the first joint attacked. Many noted physicians since that time have included the diagnosis of gout in their descriptions of diseases. The English physician, Sydenham, who lived between 1624 and 1689, distinguished gout from other forms of arthritis. His description of the acute attacks obtained from personal experience is still a medical classic. It has been said that the Methuen Treaty of 1703 between Portugal and England which lowered the import duty on port wine, vastly increased the attacks of gout in Great Britain and contributed directly to the active gout and eventual death of William Pitt. It was in 1776 that the German physician Schule identified uric acid as a constituent of urine. Eleven years later its connection with gout was proved by Wollaston, an Englishman, who isolated it from gouty tophi. After only a few more years,

Forbes, another Englishman, theorized that gouty patients would show increased uric acid in the blood, but it took another half-century for this to be proved. In 1848, Garrod, also an Englishman, devised an ingenious method to determine the uric-acid content in blood. This consisted of placing a cotton thread in two or three ounces of blood drawn into a cup and leaving it there for several days. The urate crystals gradually precipitated onto the thread. From the differing amount on the thread Garrod was able to calculate surprisingly accurate values for the uric acid in the blood and to show that these were usually increased in gout. Strangely, toward the beginning of the twentieth century the disease was thought to be disappearing and the diagnosis of gout fell into disrepute. To some extent one sees residuals of this feeling even today, for a diagnosis of gout often brings an incredulous smile to the face of the patient. In the last thirty years, however, gout, along with the other rheumatic diseases, has come in for intensive study. Many of its secrets have been revealed and although many remain to be discovered we now understand enough about the disease to provide the afflicted a comfortable life—if they will follow a few basic rules.

Meanwhile, the patient can take comfort from being in good company. Alexander the Great, Louis XIV, Dr. Sydenham, Benjamin Franklin, "Mad Anthony" Wayne, Neville Chamberlain, Lloyd George and many others have suffered from acute gouty pain. Patients may draw comfort, too, from Lord Chesterfield's rather snobbish, and not entirely accurate statement, "Gout is the distemper of a gentleman; whereas the rheumatism is the distemper of a hackney-coachman or chairman, who is obliged to be out in all weathers and at all hours."

XIV The Nature of Gout

Gout affects the entire body, but manifests itself chiefly by recurring attacks of acute painful swelling in various joints. Although the great toe is the joint most commonly affected, any of them may be involved; and gout may occur without affecting the great toe. It is usually spoken of as a "metabolic disease." "Metabolism" means the chemical changes constantly going on in the body by which new tissues are built and energy produced through the absorption and assimilation of food and oxygen, during which process the worn-out tissues are broken down and waste products eliminated. It is convenient to think of the body as a power plant with the food and oxygen supplying the energy just as coal and oil are supplied to commercial plants. The body utilizes food and eliminates its waste even as the commercial power plant must get rid of its smoke and ashes. A metabolic disease is therefore one in which something has gone wrong with this chemical mechanism. It differs from an infectious disease like pneumonia, which is due to the invasion of micro-organisms, or from an allergic disease such as asthma, in which the tissues react in an abnormal way to certain foods or pollens.

Although physicians do not know all the deviations from normal which go on in the gouty patient, or all the reasons for them, nevertheless many of the important changes have been discovered.

Basically, the "metabolic defect" in gout is in the chemical mechanism by which the body handles uric acid. In some cases, too much is produced. In others, too little is eliminated. In either case, excessive uric acid collects in the tissues and circulates in the blood. To understand gout, one must therefore know something about the formation and excretion of uric acid. Actually, uric acid is a material generally considered as a waste product, but which for some reason or other is conserved to a considerable degree by the human body. It is formed as the body uses certain chemical compounds present in many of our foods, and present also in our body cells.

Most of the foods which we eat are rather complex substances. As they pass through the stomach and intestinal tract they are broken down into simple chemicals by the action of the digestive juices. These relatively simple compounds are then absorbed by the intestine into the blood stream. From them are formed (mainly in the liver) the various compounds which the body needs to produce energy and build new tissues. Furthermore, all of our body cells and tissues are constantly being broken down and replaced. This is part of the general body metabolism and continues throughout life.

Now, in the nuclei of all cells (*nuclei*—plural form of *nucleus,* meaning center) are certain substances called nucleins. Thus, as we eat foods which contain animal or plant cells, these nucleins are taken in as part of the food. It so happens that they are extremely complex substances containing many things which the body needs, including certain proteins and sugars. So far as the gouty patient is concerned, however, the important fact is that some nucleins also contain compounds which are grouped together and called *purines*. As these purines go through the metabolic process outlined, a waste product is eventually formed called *uric acid*. This is carried by the blood to the kidneys where a portion of it is eliminated. It is because this substance forms one of the chief acid constituents in the urine that it has received the name "uric acid."

One can readily see that uric acid as it circulates in the blood and is eliminated through the urine comes from two sources. The first is from the purines in the food we eat as they are broken down; this is called the "exogenous source" of uric acid. The second source is from the purines in the tissues of the patient's own body, constantly broken down as new tissues are built up. This is called the "endogenous source" of uric acid. It is also apparent that the exogenous source of the uric acid must depend somewhat on the diet, for if one takes in foods containing large amounts of purines, he will have an excess of purines to be broken down and eliminated. The endogenous source, however, remains independent of the diet.

Until very recently it was believed that these two sources of uric acid were the only ones existing. However, since the beginning of the "Atomic Age" it has been possible to do experiments which have given us evidence of another source of uric acid. By administering one of the basic chemical constituents of purine called glycine which has been "tagged" with a radioactive substance, it has been possible to follow it through the body and to note that uric acid is actually produced from it. It seems possible, too, that other substances may also be built up directly into uric acid.

Now the uric acid from these various sources is carried by the blood to the kidneys where it is filtered through the kidney into the liquid that becomes the urine. However, only a very small portion of it actually passes out with the urine. In fact, almost 90 per cent is "reabsorbed" back into the blood stream. Though the amount varies, the average person excretes about ½ gram of uric acid a day. We shall discuss this mechanism more thoroughly later on when we consider the action of some of the drugs on the passage of uric acid from the kidney.

The trouble with most gouty patients is that they form uric acid in greater quantities than do normal individuals and since their kidneys eliminate approximately the same percentage of that which is brought to them, there is constantly an increased amount of uric acid circulating in the blood. Other gouty patients, however, seem to form uric acid in normal quantities but their "uric acid clearance" is reduced; thus, they too will have excessive amounts in the blood. In its attempt to get rid of this excessive uric acid, the blood deposits those crystals in and around various joints, in certain cartilages (particularly the ears), and in other organs, often the kidneys. These deposits are called "tophi"; any one of them is spoken of as "a gouty tophus." They are often also referred to as "uratic deposits." Actually this disease has obtained its name from these deposits. The term "gout" is derived from the Latin *gutta* which implies a drop or coagulation and was so used by early physicians in an attempt to describe these gouty tophi.

It is strange that most animals are not susceptible to gout since they break uric acid down still further chemically before excreting it. This is because an enzyme known as uricase is present in the bodies of these other mammals. This enzyme oxidizes the urate to allantoin which is then broken down to urea and excreted. But man and the anthropoid apes (and, for some mysterious reason, the Dalmatian coach hound, among dogs) do not have uricase circulating in their blood. They therefore cannot negotiate this further chemical change and so are always potential gout victims. In this respect they are like birds and reptiles. Anyone who has raised large quantities of turkeys has found some of his birds developing large deposits on the joints of the feet. This also happens in domesticated pets and birds as well as the wild ones, where deformed gouty feet may at times be seen.

XV Causes of Gout

The exact cause of gout—that is to say, the reason why some people form too much uric acid from substances which have no ill effect on others, and why some people's circulating uric acid is bound so tightly that the kidneys cannot clear it, is unknown. However, some things occur in such a large number of gouty patients that they seem to be more than coincidental. These are referred to as "predisposing causes" and will be discussed here. Those factors which cause a patient with gout to develop symptoms will be discussed in another chapter.

Heredity: That gout runs in families seems well established. It is not uncommon for a patient to mention that his brother and father also have gout. Thus, some people are seemingly born with a predisposition to the disease. This is not always true, however, and many gouty patients when questioned do not know of other members of the family who actually had true gout; nor does it necessarily mean that gouty parents will always have gouty children. However, when many families of gouty patients are studied carefully one will find numerous members who show abnormalities of uric-acid metabolism.

Sex: Men far more than women are susceptible to gout. Most statistics give the relative incidence as approximately fifty cases of male gout to one of female. Yet, women do have the disease and when they do, it acts in all respects as in men. Moreover, a high percentage of women without symptoms of true gout are found to have increased amounts of uric acid in their blood.

Age: Although most common after the age of 40, gout does occur in younger people but rarely before puberty.

The Gouty Diathesis: The word diathesis is defined as "the bodily constitution or condition predisposing to a disease." Most patients who have gout are found to be heavy-set persons, somewhat overweight, with a ruddy complexion, a good disposition, and a tendency to be carefree. This is not always so, however, and gout may hit the thin, underweight, anemic type.

Since misconceptions exist, it seems important for the patient to know that certain things are *not* the cause of gout.

(1) *Contagion:* Gout is not contagious or infectious. It cannot be "caught" by coming into contact with one who has the disease.

(2) *Climate:* Patients with gout are apparently found in all areas of the world and in all climates.

(3) *Race:* Likewise, gout appears to be a universal disease, in all races.

(4) *Excess Eating and Drinking:* Food and drink excesses are not the basic cause of gout, as will be mentioned later. It is quite true that once a person has gout these factors are quite apt to produce acute attacks, but this does not occur unless the person has the basic faulty metabolism. In this respect the disease is somewhat akin to diabetes. In diabetes the eating of excess sweets does not cause the disease; but if a patient with diabetes eats sugar and starchy foods excessively, he will develop symptoms because of his basic inability to handle these foods. So, too, the gouty patient develops symptoms because his body has a basic chemical defect and cannot cope with certain foods.

XVI The Clinical Course of Gout

The Joints: As mentioned at the beginning, gout manifests itself chiefly by recurring attacks of acute painful swelling in various joints. Although, like any other disease, it may be moderate or severe and may affect different people in different ways, the following sequence of events may be thought of as characteristic.

The onset of the first attack is usually sudden and severe. Although it may be in either sex at any age, it is most likely to be noted in a man past forty. Strangely, many attacks come on in the early morning, from two to four o'clock, awakening the patient. Any joint may be involved, but the bunion joint is the most common, and will be the first affected in about half the cases. The joint swells rapidly and takes on a reddish-purple hue, which turns white on pressure. It is usually rather warm and becomes extemely painful and tender, so much so that sometimes not even the bed covers can be tolerated. Under modern treatment this painful swelling can usually be relieved after several hours, but if it is of such moderate severity that the patient does not seek medical attention, or if he happens to be where no doctor is available, the painful swelling will persist one to four days and then gradually subside. Usually the first attack will subside completely within two weeks, even if no doctor is seen. As the joint swelling goes down, the skin over the joint becomes shiny and wrinkled. After this attack the patient may be free for many months, or even for years. It would indeed be rare for a second attack of gout to occur within six months of the first, and the second attack may be delayed as much as five to ten years. Eventually, however, the second attack comes, and is somewhat similar to the first, though it may be more, or less, severe. It may last only a day or two or it may continue up to ten or fifteen days. This attack also subsides and again the patient is symptom-free. This pattern of recurring attacks may be repeated over many years. Gradually, however, the attacks become more frequent and though they may not be quite so severe they do not subside as rapidly. Furthermore, as time goes on, more than one joint may be involved, and when this is true the patient may also experience general symptoms of weakness, malaise and fever. Gradually, too, as further attacks come, some joints will not clear completely. The acute symptoms may subside but the joint will remain enlarged or deformed. Such joints usually suffer more or less continual "low grade" pain with occasional recurrences of severe pain. This is spoken of as "chronic gouty arthritis."

In discussing the acute attacks of gout, both the character of the pain and the joints affected deserve special mention. Although the severe pain with sudden onset is that which most gouty patients remember, nevertheless many attacks will occur in which the pain is moderate, or indeed only slight. Furthermore, one severe attack may be followed by another equally painful, or by a milder attack. Exactly what governs the severity of an attack is not known. Patients who are under treatment, however, and observe the treatment faithfully have few severe pains. As to particular joints affected, practically any joint in the body can be. However, usually the spine, shoulders and hips do not give painful symptoms. This is not to say, however, that they are not involved in the gouty process, for in post-mortem examinations changes are frequently found in these areas as well as in other joints where the pain was severe. It is uncommon for the small finger joints to be affected during the early stage. As noted previously, the early attacks usually affect only one joint at a time. Later, however, if the disease becomes chronic, many joints may be affected and some may never completely return to normal. It is interesting that when the elbow joint is affected the most common site is the bursa overlying the elbow, known as the olecranon bursa. "Olecranon bursitis" is usually a sign of gout, although it may also occur in rheumatoid arthritis. Why this particular bursa should be singularly affected in gout, and others rarely so, is a question not yet answered. Nor is the question of why the bunion joint is so troublesome in this disease.

Extra-Joint Manifestations: As the stage of "chronic gouty arthritis" is reached, symptoms other than those in the joints are likely to be found.

Tophi: The excess uric acid which accumulates in the body is converted into crystals of sodium biurate which accumulate in certain areas as nodular deposits, or tophi, of varying size. Although they may occur anywhere, and in severe cases of long standing may be numerous, nevertheless they are found in some areas more commonly than in others. The most frequent site is along the free edge of the ear, while many are found behind the elbow. They also form in the cartilages and capsules of joints. Frequently they may be seen in the tendon sheaths. These deposits form slowly and may frequently go unnoticed until they have attained the size of a small pea, but if a patient is suspected of gout and is examined, deposits may be found of pinhead size. Even small tophi are usually not found with the first acute attack of gouty arthritis; in fact, it may be as much as ten or twelve years after the first attack before any evidence of tophi can be found. In rare cases the deposits may attain such tremendous size as to be unsightly or to interfere with the function of the joints. Then surgical removal may be necessary. Tophi will sometimes ulcerate and the urate crystals discharge through the skin. They have a thick, chalky appearance (*tophus* comes from a Latin word which means a chalky deposit). When this chalky material is examined on a slide under a microscope and characteristic uratic crystals are seen the diagnosis is unquestioned. Occasionally when a case is not clear-cut, physicians may nick open the skin covering a suspicious tophus and examine it under the microscope in an attempt to identify urate crystals. If this can be done the diagnosis is certain, since no other known disease produces uratic deposits.

Kidney Stones: Uric-acid crystals may also precipitate from the urine and form kidney stones of varying size. When this occurs, these stones are similar in most respects to other kidney stones. However, they do not cast a shadow in routine x-rays and, consequently, can only be demonstrated by the fact that they block the excretion of certain diagnostic dyes which are injected for this purpose. The pain depends on the size and location of the stone. It may or may not pass of its own accord, or it may cause a blockage which will require surgical intervention. Considering the total number of cases of gout, however, the incidence of kidney stones is not high.

Arteriosclerosis and Heart Disease: In the past it was thought that patients with gout were particularly susceptible to heart disease and to hardening of the arteries more than the normal person. With modern methods of treatment, however, this need not occur —provided the patient is conscientious in following the regimen his physician gives hm.

Mental Symptoms: Most attacks of gout are accompanied by, or even preceded by, changes in mood, particularly depression. These may be so common in some patients that the family or business associates may sense that an attack is coming on.

Blood Abnormalities: Certain diseases affecting particularly the blood, such as leukemia and polycythemia vera (an overproduction of red cells), are frequently associated with gout. Some physicians have thought that gout, under these circumstances, is not a primary hereditary metabolic ailment but is secondary to the blood disease. Regardless of this, when gout occurs with these blood diseases it is in all respects like its other forms.

XVII Sources of Acute Attacks of Gout

Although the slowly accumulating deposits of sodium biurate previously described may eventually deform and change a joint, this accumulation alone does not explain the severe acute attacks. There is no significant increase in the circulating uric acid before, during, or after an acute attack. Apparently, then, other factors are at work which cause a sudden deposition of uric acid crystals in the joint tissues with resultant inflammation and severe pain. Although we do not know what the exact chemical changes are which bring about these acute attacks, nevertheless we do know many physical factors which may start them. It therefore behooves the patient with gout to know what these starters are and to try to avoid them. All the factors listed will not always cause attacks in every individual. Furthermore, some of them will bring on attacks at one time and not another. However, if one would be on the safe side he should avoid them all.

INJURIES

Probably the thing which most frequently causes a case of gout to flare up and become acute is injury to a joint. The injury need not be severe. A minor twist of an ankle or a knee may touch off a very severe attack of gout. Sometimes these acute attacks are treated as sprains for many years before their true nature is recognized. Two factors help in differentiating between the two. The reaction from an injury in a normal joint is usually in direct proportion to the amount of the injury. That is to say, a mild injury produces a mild reaction, and a severe one a greater reaction. In gout, on the other hand, a minor injury can produce a severe effect with much swelling, heat, redness and pain. The other factor is the time relationship. Pain and swelling due to a joint injury usually start almost immediately. In gout, however, it is not uncommon for the ill effect to be delayed twelve to thirty-six hours.

Minor injuries can seem so commonplace that the gouty patient may not appreciate their significance. Thus, a long automobile drive with constant pressure on the accelerator may precipitate an acute attack in a big toe; unusual activities associated with spring gardening or house repairing, or a lengthy round of golf after a long winter's layoff, or even stubbing a toe, may be responsible for an acute attack.

Breaking-in a pair of new shoes can start trouble. Once the shoe has been softened and bends without difficulty it can be worn quite easily, but when new and stiff, the irritation may be sufficient to initiate an attack.

OVEREATING

Directly behind injuries as a precipitating cause of gout must be listed food intake. Both the quantity and the quality are important. Patients may apparently bring on acute attacks simply by continually overeating, but of special significance is overindulgence in those foods which contain heavy amounts of purine. Most of these are the so-called "rich meats"—liver, sweetbreads, brains, steak, duck, goose, turkey. Diet is discussed fully under treatment, and foods to be avoided are listed in Appendix A. Patients should familiarize themselves with the essential facts of these diets and try to avoid the foods which contain excessive purines. Persons with gout who are notorious heavy meat-eaters and consume large quantities of steak, turkey, goose, duck, liver, brain or sweetbreads are in danger of attacks and may persistently bring on acute episodes by refusing to give up these foods. Other gouty patients may avoid these foods, but may suffer acute attacks by attending occasional parties where heavy eating is practiced. Thus, weddings, anniversary and birthday celebrations, as well as Christmas and Thanksgiving seasonal parties, are dangerous for the gouty patient. Hunters who spend a season each year hunting, when they also eat unusually heavily several days in a row, may bring on attacks. Likewise, professional and businessmen run risks when attending conferences and conventions where large luncheons and dinners are eaten day after day.

ALCOHOL

Closely allied to the excessive ingestion of food is the excessive ingestion of alcohol. Since alcohol does not contain purine and does not overload the stomach and intestinal tract as heavy meals do, its mode of action appears to be somewhat different. The reason for this is not known, but supports the statement previously made that the acute attack of gout is not entirely from purine consumption. However, excessive alcoholic intake stands close to the head of the list as a cause of acute gouty attacks. Of course, just how much alcohol is "excessive" may be hard to state precisely. However, for most patients even a slight amount seems to be too much, and those who would be sure of a comfortable life must be teetotalers.

OPERATIONS

Patients with gout are particularly prone to suffer acute attacks during the week after an operation, unless certain precautions have been taken. Almost any operation except such minor ones as the extraction of a tooth may be followed by these acute attacks. Furthermore, the particular type of anesthesia does not seem to be the determining factor, since acute attacks may come after use of any type of anesthesia, whether general, spinal or even local. Most of these attacks occur within the week after the operation. This is directly the opposite of rheumatoid arthritis where an operation usually exerts a beneficial effect lasting several weeks. It is usually safe to say that nearly all acute attacks of arthritis within the first ten days after an operation are gouty. This is so important that the patient with gout, if he finds it necessary to have an operation, should be sure to notify his surgeon that he has gout and will need special preparation. This special preparation is not too severe. It consists simply of a completely purine-free diet for five days before and five days after an operation and the taking of small doses of colchicine regularly during that time.

MEDICINES

A number of medicines may start attacks of gout and must therefore be taken with caution. These include liver extract, penicillin, vitamin B_{12}, purgatives of any sort, bile salts, occasionally insulin, and particularly the various diuretic drugs used to increase the elimination of urine during dropsical conditions. However, these medications do not always start attacks. Some of them seem to bring on attacks in one patient and not in another. Thus, if one of the drugs mentioned is indicated for some other disease which the gouty patient has, it may be necessary to give the drug, although cautiously, and even run the risk of an acute gout attack rather than miss the benefit from the medicine.

SEASON OF THE YEAR

Most gouty patients notice that their acute attacks have a tendency to recur at a certain season. This is not constant for all, but the majority recur in the spring and fall. Hence the gouty patient should know, if possible, when his attacks are most likely to occur and watch his step at that time.

STRESS (PHYSICAL AND MENTAL)

Undue physical stress, including long exposure to cold, damp and rainy weather may bring on an attack of gout. Emotional stress and sudden nervous upsets are common causes of acute attacks in susceptible persons. One of this author's patients was an Army General in a very responsible position. His wife kept colchicine constantly ready, for when pressures built up, she knew the General would have an acute attack. Another patient was a division manager for a large food chain. On three different occasions when he opened a new store he developed acute gout. The accumulated stress of dealing with real estate developers, architects, builders, food suppliers, sales clerks, etc., put our manager in bed with a swollen toe at the time of the Grand Opening!

Although it may not be possible always to avoid these, the patient with gout should do his utmost to keep such stress to a minimum. In this same category should be mentioned that some younger gouty patients note the occurrence of acute attacks following sexual excess. This does not mean that sexual intercourse is harmful in gout. But the occasional excesses, like those of food and drink, may prove troublesome.

XVIII   The Prognosis in Gout

Physicians often speak of the "prognosis" of a disease, meaning the long-range forecast of how the patient and his disease will be at a future time. For gout the prognosis depends largely on the patient and how closely he is willing to follow the prescribed regimen.

Since the actual cause of gout is not known, it is not surprising that we have no cure. We do not yet know how to alter the basic underlying metabolic defect. Nevertheless, the disease can be controlled. Indeed, it seems safe to say that in gout more than in any other rheumatic disease (and indeed probably as much as in any chronic physical ailment), the patient's future is in his own hands. If he chooses to follow the treatment regimen closely, he will lead a comfortable life interrupted only occasionally by acute attacks and his life span need not differ from what it would be if he were free from gout. On the other hand, if he ignores the measures which it is known help control the disease, he will in all probability suffer repeated attacks and may eventually become a chronic gouty invalid.

Of course there are individual variations, or individual degrees of severity of the disease. One person may be a severe case and another a mild one. The latter may be able to break rules and have fewer attacks than would be expected. Here again, the likeness to diabetes is evident. A mild diabetic may eat certain amounts of sweets without serious results, whereas the severe diabetic will be in trouble with the slightest deviation from his diet or insulin dose. Unfortunately, our blood studies in gout are not as accurate and dependable as they are in diabetes. However, when the blood levels of uric acid remain high, the gouty patient is probably in for trouble. Conversely, when it drops promptly under treatment, the outlook is usually good.

Although the patient who ignores the treatment precautions is in for trouble, disastrous effects may not always be noted with the first break in treatment. A patient under treatment for months, or years, and getting along well may decide to ignore the rules "just once" and enjoy a party with a lot of drinking and heavy eating. If he has no ill effects he decides that he is getting along quite well, or may even think his gout is cured. This feeling is heightened when he indulges in a second, and possibly a third or fourth party without serious result; but sooner or later the parties catch up with him and he suffers a severe, and possibly prolonged attack, which is difficult to control. Furthermore, he may develop certain tophi in the joints or other tissues during this apparently innocuous period and his setback may be irreversible. The situation is somewhat like disciplining a small child. He is told that if he eats green apples he will develop a stomach-ache, but he eats one or two without developing any symptoms and so on some occasion sits down to enjoy a real feast. Then he learns the truth of the Scriptural passage, "Be sure your sins will find you out."

In view of these facts the gouty patient should realize that he must keep his disease under control during his entire lifetime. The treatment is a nuisance and sometimes an inconvenience, but after all it is not too drastic. The human body is subject to many ills and many woes, and gout is not the worst.

XIX Laboratory Tests

As mentioned in chapter XII, laboratory tests are not infallible in the rheumatic diseases. This is particularly true of gout. But certain ones are of great significance.

Identification of Gouty (Sodium Biurate) Crystals: If material from a discharging gouty tophus is spread thinly on a microscope slide and then examined under a high-power miscroscope, typical sodium biurate crystals can be identified. If a swelling near a joint or on a fold of the ear is suspected of being a tophus, but does not discharge, material from the area can be obtained and checked on the microscopic slide. Tophi invariably contain crystals and these can nearly always be obtained and identified if a proper search is made.

Likewise, when fluid is taken from a joint swollen by an acute attack of gout, it will be found to contain typical crystals of sodium biurate. These can usually be identified by direct examination under the microscope. If there is any question, polarized light will settle it. This is particularly helpful when true gout must be distinguished from "pseudo-gout" (chrondrocalcinosis) — a disease which may mimic gout. In this latter condition, the crystals which are seen in the fluid are those of calcium and do not shine in the polarized light as do the gouty crystals.

Blood Uric Acid: Since the gouty patient is accumulating increased amounts of uric acid, this is usually reflected in the blood where higher concentrations are found. Sometimes during the early stages of the disease, this is not true, but as gout progresses, an elevated uric acid is almost always present. The normal individual will rarely exceed 6 milligrams of uric acid per 100 cubic centimeters of blood unless he is taking a medication which causes the body to retain uric acid. Most gouty patients will have a reading of 7-9. For some strange reason, it is extremely rare for it ever to rise above ten, regardless of the severity of the condition or its duration. The ratios of uric acid will usually drop under proper treatment. Yet they do not seem to be altered before, during or after an acute attack. However, a patient who has had his gout under control with a normal blood content of uric acid, and then begins to ignore treatment, may show a rise in the blood uric acid, and this usually means impending trouble. As more accurate methods of measuring the circulating uric acid are developed, the usefulness of this test may be greatly increased. It seems logical to believe that our tests of today are not critical enough to register slight variations and that these variations may be significant.

X-ray: In the early stages of gout, joints appear perfectly normal by x-ray. As time goes on, however, cartilage may be destroyed. Sodium biurate may be deposited in the bone below the articulating surface and then x-rays of any joint may show much deformity. The changes, however, are not characteristic and a diagnosis of gout can rarely be made from the x-ray picture alone.

XX   Treatment

A review of its clinical course shows that gout may be divided into two distinct phases. The first phase is that of the acute attack, during which one or more joints are painful and swollen. The other phase might be called the quiescent or interval phase, during which the patient is apparently normal but during which excessive uric acid is building up in his body and depositing in tissues where it should not be. Treatment therefore also may be conveniently divided into two separate regimens. The first is in the acute attack, when the aim is to relieve the patient of the acute pain and disability. The second phase of treatment is the "interval regimen," during which an attempt is made to prevent the excess accumulation of uric acid. It is usually the acute attack which brings the patient to the physician, and the pain may be so severe that the sufferer is willing to submit to almost anything to obtain relief. During the quiescent phase, without any painful reminder of the damage going on in his body he is likely to become careless; yet treatment during this time is by far the more important, so far as the eventual outcome of the disease is concerned, for if the uric acid can be controlled, serious deformities will not result. It will therefore be discussed first.

PART I. INTERVAL REGIMEN

Since gout is due to the excess production of uric acid and its decreased elimination, it logically follows that the way to treat the disease is to see to it that the body takes in as small amounts as possible of those materials used in the formation of the uric acid, and then try to force a greater elimination of uric acid than the gouty patient normally is capable of doing. The former is accomplished through dietary control and the latter through certain drugs. It is important to remember the statement made earlier in this manual that the severity of the gouty process differs from one patient to another. Thus, it may be important for one person to be very rigid in his control, whereas the patient with milder gout may "get by" with fewer restrictions.

Dietary Treatment: Since uric acid is formed from purines, the basis of the dietary treatment must be the restriction of those foods which contain purines. These are listed in detail in Appendix A in the back of this manual, and the gouty patient should keep this list handy until he has familiarized himself with it. The chief offending foods are easily remembered. Meats are the highest of all in purines. Particularly is this true of the glandular meats, such as liver, kidneys, brains and sweetbreads; steak is also high in purine content. Since uric acid is excreted more readily when the fat in the diet is restricted, the fatty meats such as goose, duck, squab, turkey and pork must also be thought of as offending agents. Following the meats come the whole-grain cereals and a few vegetables: beans (navy, kidney or lima), asparagus, cauliflower, mushrooms, onions and peas. Meat extracts and gravies are also taboo.

Because of the "low-fat rule" which limits fats because of their interference with the elimination of uric acid, pastries, pies, ice cream, and nuts must also be taken in limited quantities. Alcohol, though it contains no purine, must be completely eliminated from the diet because of its tendency to bring on acute attacks.

This then is the negative side of the diet, and although these foods may be permitted to a certain extent, they should be drastically reduced. The positive side of the diet—that is to say, those foods which will be relied on chiefly to supply the necessary nourishment—will then include vegetables (other than those listed), cereals (except whole grain), breads (except whole wheat and pumpernickel), fruits, milk, cheese, eggs and butter in limited quantities.

Coffee, Tea, Cocoa and Soft Drinks: It was formerly thought that these drinks should be prohibited on a gouty diet, but more recent tests indicate that they are permissible if the calories they contain do not raise the total calories above the limit the patient is allowed.

During the quiescent interval it seems a good plan to set aside two days a week for a "purine-free" diet and to keep the diet on the other days of the week a "low-purine" scale. To prevent a patient from forgetting his two days without purines, it is usually advisable to set aside the same two days each week. The plan does not have to be too rigid, however, and if one goes visiting on what is usually a "purine-free day," he may in deference to his host wish to change this with one of the "low-purine days."

In addition to the type of food, the amount must be considered. Many gouty patients are overweight and must reduce. This should never be done rapidly, as sudden marked weight loss may cause an acute attack. A 1,200-calorie diet per day is usually a good average when a person is trying to reduce. For the average working man the diet will contain 2,000 to 2,400 calories. Sample menus are included in Appendix A. In these menus Wednesday and Friday have been designated "purine-free days" and on these days cheese, eggs and milk replace meat and fish. A convenient check list of foods for gouty patients is also included.

Drug Therapy: In addition to limiting the intake of purines, to hold the formation of uric acid to a minimum, treatment during the quiescent phase must include the use of some drug to help eliminate more uric acid than would be done normally. Such a drug is called "a uricosuric agent," and the increased uric-acid elimination it produces is spoken of as the "uricosuric effect." For years physicians have known that such drugs existed. Cinchophen and massive doses of aspirin (eighteen to twenty tablets per day) were the most commonly used. But these had distinct disadvantages. Cinchophen sometimes damaged the liver, and such large doses of aspirin caused stomach upset and ringing in the ears. But intensive searches have been made to develop an effective uricosuric drug without significant side reactions. Several such drugs are now available.

Probenecid (Benemid): This drug has been commercially available since about 1950 and has, therefore, had adequate time to prove its usefulness. It exerts a strong uricosuric effect, which does not appear to be lost over a long-continued administration, and serious side reactions are very rare. Furthermore, only one or two tablets per day are usually adequate. When the drug is first started there may be a tendency for a mild gouty flare-up, and for this reason some colchicine is often prescribed along with Benemid during the first few weeks. The administration of this former drug is described more completely under the treatment of the acute attack.

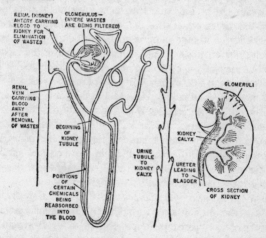

FIGURE 15

To understand how probenecid acts one must understand something of the anatomy and physiology of the kidney, for it is in the kidney that the uric acid is extracted from the blood and passed out into the urine. If one cuts a kidney open and examines it with a hand glass, the outer half of the kidney along its curved border will be seen to contain small round areas resembling pinheads (Figure 15). These are called "glomeruli" and if examined under a microscope they have the appearance of whirled balls of cotton. When they are dissected out, stained, and examined under extremely high power, it is seen that the whirled portion of each glomerulus is composed of two distinct tubes lying close together and intimately related. One of these is a tiny blood vessel and as the blood passes through it, water and certain chemicals pass through the very thin wall into the other, which is the beginning of the urine tube. As the whirls straighten out, the blood vessel and the urine tube still lie close together and are grouped together at the central portion of the kidney, giving the appearance there, when examined by the hand lens, of many straight lines pointing toward the center crescent of the kidney. In this tubulous portion of the kidney a strange thing is going on. Some of the chemicals originally filtered from the blood into the urine in the glomerulus are being reabsorbed back into the blood. Although this at first seems strange, it is nevertheless part of nature's delicately balanced method for retaining the exact constituents such as sugar and proteins in the blood, and removing only the excess for discard through the urine. As the kidney tubes get larger, the blood vessels branch away from them and return to the blood system. The kidney tubes on the other hand join together, and finally form the large tube which leads from the kidney down to the bladder carrying the urine for excretion from the body.

Now, uric acid participates in this "filter—reabsorption" process. A large quantity of it is filtered through the glomerulus, but most of it is reabsorbed into the blood in the tubule. Probenecid has the power to decrease some of this reabsorption into the tubule. Thus when it is being taken, instead of the usual 90 per cent of that which is filtered through the kidney glomerulus being reabsorbed, only about 80 per cent is. The gouty patient taking probenecid, therefore, excretes about twice as much uric acid in a day as he does without the drug. Moreover, this action is accomplished without any deleterious effect on the kidney.

Many patients take probenecid indefinitely without evidence of any unpleasant side or toxic effects.

Although the amount of uric acid excreted is double that when probenecid is not taken, there is still a great deal circulating in the blood. It is therefore quite obvious that it will require some time to eliminate a large quantity of uric acid from the body. But with careful blood examinations for uric acid, it is evident that this falls at a fairly rapid rate toward the normal, and furthermore, as a patient continues to take an active uricosuric agent, the large deposits of urate in the body (the tophi) may be gradually broken down and excreted. Thus many patients under continuous probenecid therapy report that their tophi shrink in size and some disappear completely. This same beneficial effect may even be noted in the bone where x-rays may show the decrease of uratic deposits with the re-formation of normal bone. The length of time necessary for such a process depends on the size of the deposit and the constant adherence to the regimen.

Phenylbutazone (Butazolidin): This drug, which was previously described as useful in other forms of arthritis, has also been found to be an active uricosuric agent. Since it may, at times, produce toxic reactions it is less popular than probenecid. However, occasionally patients seem intolerant of the latter and then phenylbutazone is an effective substitute.

Anturane: This drug is a derivative of phenylbutazone and it, too, exerts a uricosuric effect like phenylbutazone. However, it also may have toxic side reactions although these are rare.

Griseofulvin: This drug, which is used primarily in the treatment of fungus infections (as athlete's foot), also exerts a strong uricosuric effect. The daily cost, however, is considerably higher than the other drugs and for this reason it is seldom used for this purpose.

Allopurinol (Zyloprim): This drug acts in an entirely different way to lower the concentration of uric acid found circulating in the blood. Indeed, it has no action on the excretion of the uric acid; it interrupts the "metabolic breakdown" of purines before they reach the stage of uric acid. A full discussion of this would involve more organic chemistry that is necessary for the reader to be burdened with. But, if he is interested in big words, he might like to know that substances called xanthine and hypoxanthine are formed from purines, and uric acid in turn is formed from these. Now, allopurinol comes into the picture by preventing this final step in the metabolic pathway. The body then seems to be able to eliminate these compounds and spare the gouty patient the insult of the excessive uric acid production.

Occasionally when patients first start a uricosuric agent, they may develop acute attacks which are rather surprising and discouraging. This is a temporary situation, however, and probably due to certain "mobilizing" of the uric acid in the system. Furthermore, these attacks are usually very easily controlled by the administration of colchicine as mentioned. After the patient has been under treatment for some weeks he may reasonably expect to have fewer and fewer attacks.

Fluid Intake: In a previous chapter, it was mentioned that some patients with gout will develop kidney stones containing uric acid crystals. The best way to prevent their formation is to keep the urine diluted by drinking copious quantities of water. Three quarts a day is the desired goal. This much water may be hard to "get down," but to be on the safe side, two quarts is a minimum for all gouty patients.

Summary: One may therefore summarize the interval treatment of gout during the quiescent phase as follows:

1. Restriction of the diet, to avoid eating foods containing purines which can increase the formation of uric acid in the body.
2. Taking a drug which helps the body put out more uric acid than it normally would do, or one that keeps the body from breaking down its purines to uric acid.
3. Drinking at least two quarts of water per day.
4. Alkalinizing the urine in persons who have developed stones in the past.
5. The careful avoidance of those factors which could produce an acute attack.

PART II. TREATMENT IN
THE ACUTE ATTACK

The chief aim of treatment during an acute attack is to relieve as rapidly as possible the severe pain and swelling which the patient is experiencing. This is best accomplished by certain drug therapy.

Colchicine: The value of this drug in relieving acute upsets of gout has been known for centuries. It is derived from the autumn-flowering plant, *Colchicum autumnale*, also known as the fall saffron or autumn crocus. Colchicum was so named by the ancient Greeks because it flourished in Colchio in Asia Minor. It is believed that references in one of the ancient Egyptian manuscripts known as the "Ebers Papyrus," prepared in 1,500 B.C., is to a drug identical with or similar to colchicine. It is known to have been used by a physician of Constantinople, Jacques Psychriste, in the time of Emperor Leo the Great, A.D. 457-474, and by Alexander of Tralles, during the sixth century, and was recommended by the medical school of Salerno in the twelfth century. Although it fell into disrepute about the seventeenth century, it was revived in the eighteenth and has been used ever since. Most of the drug used for American supplies comes from Holland, Italy or Yugoslavia. The drug colchicine is almost unique in medicine in that it is used in only one disease—gout—yet in that disease is rapidly and universally effectual. This is so true that "the colchicine test" is sometimes used to determine whether a swollen joint is actually gouty or not. If it responds to colchicine it is assumed the swelling is from gout; if not, other causes are usually sought. (Except in long-standing chronic gouty arthritis which may become resistant to colchicine.) It is also of interest that, although colchicine has only this single usefulness in medicine, it is used extensively in plant breeding and studies of genetics, since it has the power of doubling chromosomes.

The exact mode of action by which colchicine stops the acute attack is not certain. However, it appears to interfere with the destruction of uric acid crystals by the white cells. It thus stops the production of lactic acid which occurs as those cells are broken down and consequently reduces the inflammation. Other mechanisms as yet unknown may be taking place.

Colchicine is usually prescribed in tablet form, each containing either 1/100 or 1/120 of a grain. Formerly the wine of colchicum was used but because this is unstable and the concentration varies as time goes on, the tablets, which are quite stable, are now preferred. The actual mode of administration will vary, but the most common program is to start with two tablets and then to take one additional tablet every hour through the day until the pain is relieved or intestinal symptoms develop. This is usually a total of six to nine tablets. Thus, about four or five hours after the drug is begun the patient is conscious that there is less tension in the joint, the swelling is beginning to subside, and the pain is relieved. About this same time there are usually intestinal symptoms, with loosening of the bowels and on occasion even marked diarrhea. The number of tablets that will produce these changes is referred to as "the diarrheal dose." The therapeutically effective dose is ordinarily one or two tablets less than the "diarrheal dose," and thus if a patient develops diarrhea, he should jot down the number of tablets he has taken and on any subsequent administration take one or two less. It is usually wise to continue colchicine for about a week. After the first day, one tablet three times a day for a week is usually enough to insure against recurrence of the acute attack. Some patients, however, find that this too will precipitate intestinal symptoms and the dose must be decreased, in some cases to as little as one tablet every other day.

Patients with gout should maintain on hand a supply of colchicine, for oftentimes they are able to tell when an attack is starting. At such times two or three tablets a day for three or four days may prevent the attack from ever becoming serious.

In some patients the intestinal symptoms developing under colchicine may be so severe that it cannot be tolerated. Then the drug may be administered intravenously. Indeed, some physicians prefer to use this method exclusively. It has the disadvantage that it must be given in the physician's office. Furthermore, some patients object to a needle, although most people prefer this to repeated tablets with the possibility of stomach upset.

ACTH: ACTH is a most effective drug in stopping the acute gouty attacks. A single dose often brings relief in a few hours, especially in early cases. However, the attack may recur twenty-four hours later, and for this reason colchicine in moderate doses is usually continued for about a week after the dose of ACTH. Paradoxically, ACTH has been known to cause acute attacks of gout. It has been suggested that these factors may give a clue as to the chemical mechanism which normally precedes an acute attack. Since corticotropin is a normal secretion of the pituitary gland which stimulates the cortex of the adrenal gland to produce cortisone, it may well be that the various factors listed previously in this outline as immediate causes of an acute attack set up a sudden stimulation of ACTH production with a primary increase in cortisone and then a compensatory drop in cortisone, thus leading to an acute attack. Whether this is true or whether the entire mechanism is temporarily paralyzed is not yet known; but from a therapeutic view, the prompt administration of ACTH does usually check an attack.

Phenylbutazone: This drug has been shown to have a prompt action in relieving the acute phase of gout. It may be administered either by mouth or by intramuscular injection. However, tests have shown that it is absorbed from the intestinal tract as rapidly as it is from the tissues; hence it is now almost always given by mouth. Eight hundred milligrams is the amount which is usually necessary to relieve an acute attack. This is usually given two tablets (100 mgm each) every hour for a total of four doses. In the majority of cases this will terminate an attack in twenty-four hours. In some cases, however, it may be necessary to administer additional phenylbutazone for one or two days extra.

It will be recalled that phenylbutazone, like probenecid, will also lower the blood uric acid through its uricosuric effect. This drug, therefore, has the advantage of stopping the acute attacks and also of lowering the concentration of uric acid in the blood. A single tablet may, therefore, replace a combination of colchicine and probenecid during the interval treatment. However, as previously noted, phenylbutazone, unfortunately, produces toxic symptoms in some patients. These include stomach upset (with occasional reactivation of peptic ulcer), skin rashes, elevation of blood pressure and depression of the blood count. Although not too common, these unpleasant side reactions occur frequently enough to require caution in the use of the drug.

Indomethacin (Indocin): This has also been found useful in relieving the acute attacks of gout. Two to six capsules may be needed in patients who are responsive to this medicine. Attacks may be aborted within two to three hours. Toxic symptoms, similar to those noted above under phenylbutazone, may at times be noted by patients taking indomethacin. Its use also must be carefully watched by a physician.

The foregoing drugs have been recommended as useful in relieving acute attacks of gout. Each will usually do this quite promptly in the early stages. However, after numerous attacks have occurred and the late stage of the disease has set in, to relieve the recurring acute attacks is more difficult. It is not uncommon for a man who has had numerous mildly acute attacks involving only a single joint and who has always obtained relief from colchicine, to get careless about his interval regimen and neglect the specified diet. Sooner or later this man may develop a severe attack involving several joints at the same time and find that the colchicine which he has previously taken is no longer effective. He may feel that he has developed some new disease, but it is only a new phase of the old. It is in such attacks that intravenous colchicine and ACTH have their greatest use, for with the combination of the two, even the most stubborn acute attack in a chronic case can usually be brought under control within four or five days.

Other Measures to Be Followed During the Acute Attack: During the acute attack the patient should rest in bed, since physical activity apparently increases the severity of the attack and makes it last longer. Furthermore, moist compresses over the affected joint are usually useful in relieving the pain. Most patients prefer these compresses warm, but others find that ice packs are of greater benefit. This can be determined only by trial and error. At such times the diet should also be completely purine-free. Should the attack be unusually severe, narcotics, perhaps small doses of codeine, Demerol, or Dolophine may be prescribed by the physician.

It should be emphasized that after a uricosuric agent such as probenecid has been started, it too should be continued through the acute attack in addition to the measures outlined. Since colchicine does not increase uric-acid elimination, discontinuing the uricosuric agent even during a short period would permit some increase in the uric-acid level of the blood and so retard some of the previously attained progress.

PART III. OPERATIONS

As mentioned previously, a patient with gout is prone to suffer a severe acute attack immediately after an operation or administration of an anesthetic. Since, however, a gout patient is subject to all the ills that a normal person is, operations may at times be necessary. If the operation can be anticipated, the patient should be on a purine-free diet five days before and five days after the operation. In addition, he should take three tablets of colchicine daily during this period. If an emergency operation is necessary and the preparation cannot be accomplished beforehand, the purine-free diet and colchicine should be started immediately afterward. If the patient is not permitted anything by mouth for several days after the operation, the colchicine may be given intravenously.

XXI   Quackery and Arthritis

*Take a garlick, two cloves, of gum, ammonia, one
drachm, blend them, by bruising, together; make
them into two or three bolusses, with fair water,
and swallow them, one at night and one in the
morning. Drink, while taking this recipe, sassafras tea, made very strong, so as to have the
tea pot filled with the chips.*

According to the Virginia Gazette of April 9, 1767, the
above

*is generally found to banish the rheumatism and
even contractions in the joints, in a few times
taking. It is very famous in America, and a
hundred pounds have been given for the recipe.*

Sounds silly does it not? But it is no more foolish than wearing
copper bracelets in the hope of relieving arthritis, and many sup-
posedly intelligent people have succumbed to such fanciful thinking.
In fact, an elderly patient of mine has been wearing one for over
ten years because she promised her husband on his death bed
that she would. He had read of this "cure" in a book on folklore
and had purchased a bracelet the day before he had a fatal heart
attack. It apparently has not done much good for she comes to
my office about every two or three months to get her painful joints
and back injected. But she is not alone—for The Arthritis Foundation estimates that $400,000,000 is spent every year on fake
"remedies"—medicines and gadgets that have no value. Indeed, at
times, such things may be worse than worthless for patients may

delay seeking competent advice while wasting time on nostrums. Federal agents of the Food and Drug Administration and the Federal Trade Commission are kept busy trying to apprehend the quacks who prey on a gullible public with their spurious products.

Alfalfa tea became popular some years ago and was widely publicized as "God's green herb" by a quack who placed the title "Rev." before his name. He founded "The Society of Good Samaritans"—dues for which were $17.00 each three months. Persons belonging to the society were mailed "free" (when their dues were paid, of course) sufficient alfalfa to "treat" their arthritis during the three month period. Since the total cost of the alfalfa and the mailings was less than $3.00, the "reverend" was doing all right by himself—until the F.D.A. cracked down after scientifically controlled tests showed it to be no good.

An interesting side light on this man's operation was provided in some of his literature. God's green herb, he wrote, was often robbed of its life-giving properties by improper fertilization during cultivation. So his followers were advised to use only that which he furnished and would vouch for. But government agents found he was buying alfalfa seed on the open market and had no idea where or how it had been cultivated.

"Super" aspirins are constantly being marketed with wild and extravagant claims. We have mentioned previously that aspirin is an excellent medicine in the treatment of most forms of rheumatism. But some manufacturers often add small amounts of materials that have little or no extra benefits, charge many times what the aspirin is worth, and sell the product through false or misleading claims. I have, in my files, a letter from the president of such a company in which he threatens to hold me responsible for loss of revenue for any false statements I might make about his products. It was one which contained a small amount of a calcium product in addition to about four grains of aspirin. Our tests at the Georgetown Rheumatology Clinic showed that the drug had no value over plain aspirin (but sold for $2.00 per 100 tablets). Those tests were corroborated in another clinic and the government forced the manufacturer to alter his advertisements.

My article reporting our findings was published in a medical journal and the letter I mentioned arrived shortly thereafter.

We also worked with the Federal agencies in showing that a popular mineral water was no better than ordinary tap water as a treatment.

In testing both of these products, we used what is known as a "double blind technic." The Food and Drug Administration furnished us the products to be tested and an alternate product which looked just like it but had a different label on the bottle. In the case of the super aspirin tested, the alternate product was plain aspirin of a strength identical to that of the tested tablet. In the case of the mineral water, it was an identical bottle filled with water from the city supply. Neither the doctors in the clinic nor the patients in the test knew which was which until the test was over and the reports filed. Hence, there was no partisanship for or against the product during the test.

As noted under our previous discussion of diet, various foods and combination have been promoted as beneficial to arthritis. These are usually recommended in books or by lectures. Cod liver oil and orange juice, honey and vinegar, and "immune" milk have all been thoroughly investigated and shown to have no value in the treatment of arthritis. Yet, each has been highly recommended and widely publicized as curative. Condensed sea water has been sold to the unwary for as high as $3.00 a pint—it is useless!

Of far more serious concern, however, are potent drugs which have been purchased by American arthritics in neighboring countries. The most notable of these is a drug developed several years ago by a physician in Canada who previously had been selling a special hair tonic he made in his basement. Because its principal ingredient is a cortisone-like drug, patients with arthritis show immediate improvement when starting the drug. And since the exact formula is kept secret, patients believe they are receiving a new miracle drug. Despite an urgent plea from the Medical Director of the Arthritis Foundation, a national magazine made this remedy its feature story of the week several years ago.

Thousands of persons flocked to Canada. They purchased the drug and returned taking it without supervision and with inevitable results. Despite the developer's claims that hormones in the drug prevent side reaction, all the unpleasant complications of cortisone still appear. At least three persons taking the drug have died. It is a dangerous remedy.

In addition to worthless and dangerous drugs, arthritis sufferers are often victimized by promoters of useless gadgets and devices. One of these was a single electric bulb and a lamp shade. Affected joints were "treated" by being bathed in a blue light which came from a blue piece of plastic over the bulb. Its benefit was no greater than that obtained from the heat of any light bulb costing a fraction of the fancy one. But electricity seems to hold a special attraction for the originators of these things. The "Inducto-scope" had coils of electric wire into which the part to be treated was inserted. The Z-ray (at $50.00) claimed to "expand the arteries" of the victim and so make him overcome his arthritis. Neither had any therapeutic value. Quacks are particularly quick to exploit new and popular scientific discoveries. Shortly after the explosion of the first atom bomb, uranium treatments were recommended. People were charged $10.00 to sit in the ore-lined rooms of old mine tunnels. And a "Wonder Glove," allegedly lined with uranium ore sold for $100.00. It was absolutely useless as a treatment for arthritis.

So we might go on until we filled up a whole book. And the questions that many readers will ask is, "How come people throw away such money?" 'Why aren't they warned?" And the answer is, "They are—but refuse to listen." The American Medical Association has a whole section devoted to investigating frauds. Several government agencies do too—primarily the Federal Trade Commission and the Food and Drug Administration. The Arthritis Foundation helps in publicizing fakes and quacks. But then Barnum was right, "The public likes to be fooled." Remember Krebiozen—the cancer "cure"? Millions of dollars were spent by unwary victims and when the American Medical Association warned against the drug, it was villified and accused of trying to block the sale of a life-saving drug. Imagine! Even a distinguished U.S. Senator joined the attack against organized medicine. Finally, the National Institute of Health had to act as referee. Their scientists reviewed 100 cases which the distributors of Krebiozen claimed had been cured by the drug. The result: not one case of cancer had been cured. Many had died from the spread of the disease. And when a young chemist finally broke the secret formula, it turned out to be an innocuous compound found in everyone's body—each $7.00 ampule contained less than 10c worth of material!

Unfortunately, some editors think more of their circulation than they do of their reader's health. The editor of that magazine which published the article on the Canadian drug might be so described. He had all the facts presented to him before the journal went to press. But he knew that a sensational article on a new remedy for arthritis would sell his magazine. So the warnings given were played down and made to appear as though they were just overcautious anxieties of reactionary physicians. Unfortunately, freedom of the press does not always mean honesty of the writers.

So how can the arthritic guard against such schemes? There are a few rules:

1. Be suspicious of anyone—physician or layman—who promises a sure cure. Much can be done to relieve and often arrest the disease, but just now, a cure does not exist.

2. Be suspicious of anyone who has a "secret" formula— particularly one which is claimed to have recently been brought from abroad. Remember that every bona fide medical discovery is announced widely in medical journals throughout the world.

3. Do not be fooled by testimonials. Many of these come from patients who never had true arthritis—others are due to spontaneous remissions—many are deliberate falsehoods.

4. Be wary of devices which are claimed to provide more than temporary relief.

If in doubt, ask your physician or write to:

The Medical Director
The Arthritis Foundation
Avenue of the Americas
New York City

A six-cent stamp may save you many dollars and much discomfort.

XXII Conclusion

This, then, is the story of arthritis, rheumatism and gout as we know it today. Like so many things in life, part of it is discouraging, part encouraging; and which of the two predominates—whether the patient shall have the disease or the disease shall have him—depends on the patient's attitude, and how closely he follows the necessary regimen.

Possibly the most encouraging factor in the whole situation is that this book might become obsolete tomorrow. The interest of laymen and physicians mentioned in the Introduction is on the increase; each year sees vital new discoveries. It is not at all beyond the realm of possibility that, fairly soon, the basic defects in many of the conditions will have been identified and effective remedies made available.

Meanwhile, it behooves the rheumatic patient to walk rigidly in the strait and narrow way that leads to his medical salvation. In the last analysis, it is up to you!

PART THREE

Appendix A: Diets

On the following pages are listed a variety of diets which the arthritic and gouty patient will find useful. All have been carefully prepared to supply the daily requirements of vitamins and minerals. At the top of each diet is listed its caloric content and general indication. All may be supplemented by the additional use of gelatin taken either with or between meals, to increase the total daily protein. Persons on a reducing diet may have only two envelopes per day, others may use up to six or eight. Medical supervision in the selection of the proper diet is essential.

DIET I

APPROXIMATELY 2,400 CALORIES
WITH 100 GRAMS PROTEIN

This is an average diet for a person of normal weight, doing moderate physical work.

MEAL PLAN

Breakfast

Juice or fruit, preferably citrus
Cereal with milk and sugar
2 eggs, any style
1 slice toast with butter
Milk, 8 ounces
Coffee or tea, cream and sugar if desired

Lunch

Sandwich
    2 slices of bread with butter or mayonnaise
    2 ounces meat or substitute (*See* page 148)
    lettuce

Raw vegetables if desired, such as lettuce, celery and carrot sticks, radishes, tomatoes, etc.

Dessert—sweet dessert such as pie or cake or fresh or canned fruit

Milk, 8 ounces

Coffee or tea, cream and sugar if desired

Dinner

5 ounces meat or substitute (*See* below)

Potato

Cooked vegetable

Salad, fruit or vegetable

1 slice bread with butter

Dessert—sweet dessert such as pie or cake or fresh or canned fruit
(Limit choice of sweet dessert to once daily)

Milk, 8 ounces

Coffee or tea, cream and sugar if desired

The following will supply 2 ounces of meat or its equivalent:

A) 2 slices of cold cuts
B) 2 frankfurters
C) ½ cup of salmon, tuna or crabmeat
D) 12 medium sardines
E) 2 slices cheddar or American cheese
F) ½ cup cottage cheese
G) 2 eggs
H) 4 tablespoons peanut butter
I) 1 medium slice of meat or poultry

The following will supply 5 ounces of meat or its equivalent:

A) 5 ounces of fish
B) 2 large veal or pork loin chops
C) 3 large lamb chops
D) 2 slices, each approximately 4" x 2½" x ½" of a roast, steak, or poultry

Assistance with estimation of meat weights may be obtained from your butcher or by noting weights on labels of pre-packaged meats. If a bedtime feeding is desired, part of the dinner meal may be reserved, such as the milk and dessert or bread (crackers may be substituted for the bread).

SAMPLE MENUS OF DIET I

Choice No. 1

Breakfast

Orange juice
Cereal
Two fried eggs
Buttered toast
Milk
Coffee or tea, cream and sugar

Lunch

Hamburger on bun or 2 frankfurters on bun
Coleslaw
Apple pie
Milk
Coffee or tea, if desired

Dinner

2 baked pork chops
Escalloped potatoes
Broccoli
Tossed vegetable salad with dressing
Bread and butter
Fruit cup
Milk
Coffee or tea, if desired

Choice No. 2

Breakfast

½ Grapefruit
2 soft-cooked eggs
2 slices buttered toast
Milk
Coffee or tea, cream and sugar

Lunch

Sandwich
    2 slices bread
    1 slice cold cut and 1 slice cheese
    butter or mayonnaise
    lettuce
Apple
Milk
Coffee or tea, cream and sugar

Dinner

Pot roast of beef (5 ounces)
Baked potato
Carrots
Mixed fruit salad
Bread and butter
Rice pudding
Milk
Coffee or tea, cream and sugar

Choice No. 3

Breakfast

Stewed prunes
Ham or Canadian bacon (2 ounces)
2 slices buttered toast
Milk
Coffee or tea, cream and sugar

Lunch

Cottage cheese (about ½ cup) with a tossed vegetable salad
2 small dinner rolls with butter
Orange
Milk
Coffee or tea, cream and sugar

Dinner

Italian spaghetti with meat sauce and meat balls (2 large or 3 small)
Chef's salad
Bread sticks
Jello
Milk
Coffee or tea, cream and sugar

DIET II
APPROXIMATELY 4,000 CALORIES
WITH 130 GRAMS PROTEIN

This diet is for underweight persons who are attempting to increase weight.

In order to insure an intake of 4,000 calories, care should be taken to use liberally food such as butter or margarine, oils, shortenings, cream, mayonnaise and sugar.

Meats may be prepared in any way—boiled, broiled, baked, fried, etc.

MEAL PLAN

Breakfast

Large glass fruit juice or sweetened fruit
Cereal with cream and sugar
One egg with ham or Canadian bacon or 2 eggs
2 slices buttered toast and jelly
Large glass of milk and cream mixed
Coffee or tea, cream and sugar

Lunch

2 sandwiches, each to consist of 2 slices bread, butter and/or mayonnaise, 2 ounces meat or substitute (*See* page 148)
Raw vegetables as desired
Dessert, preferably a sweet one such as pie, cake, pudding, etc.
Large glass milk and cream mixed
Coffee or tea, cream and sugar

Dinner

5 ounces meat or substitute (*See* page 148)
Potato
Cooked vegetable
Fruit or vegetable salad
1 slice bread with butter
Dessert, preferably a sweet one such as pie, cake, pudding, etc.
Large glass milk and cream mixed
Coffee or tea, cream and sugar

Bedtime

Sandwich: 2 slices bread, butter and/or mayonnaise, 2 ounces meat or
   substitute (*See* page 148)
Large glass milk and cream mixed

SAMPLE MENUS OF DIET II

Choice No. 1

Breakfast

Large glass orange juice
Oatmeal with cream and sugar
1 egg and ham
2 slices butter toast and jelly
Large glass milk and cream mixed
Coffee or tea, cream and sugar

Lunch

2 sandwiches
   a. 2 slices rye bread, 1 slice Swiss cheese and 1 slice cooked ham,
      butter and/or mayonnaise, lettuce
   b. 2 slices bread, 2 slices bologna, butter and/or mayonnaise,
      lettuce
Carrot sticks
Apple pie
Large glass milk and cream mixed
Coffee or tea, cream and sugar

Dinner

2 large baked veal chops
Baked potato with butter
Brussels sprouts
Waldorf salad
Bread with butter and jelly
Fudge pudding with whipped cream
Large glass milk and cream mixed
Coffee or tea, cream and sugar

Bedtime

Sandwich: 2 slices bread, butter and/or mayonnaise, 2 ounces meat
   or substitute (*See* page 148)
Large glass milk and cream mixed

Choice No. 2

Breakfast

Stewed prunes
Cornflakes with cream and sugar
2 fried eggs
2 slices buttered toast with jam
Large glass milk and cream mixed
Coffee or tea, cream and sugar

Lunch

2 sandwiches
    a. 2 slices bread, 2 slices cheese, butter and/or mayonnaise, lettuce, pickles
    b. 2 slices bread, ½ cup tuna fish in tuna salad with mayonnaise
Celery sticks
Ice cream
Large glass milk and cream mixed
Coffee or tea, cream and sugar

Dinner

1 large pork chop
Whipped potatoes
Corn O'Brien
Fresh fruit salad with ½ cup cottage cheese
Bread with butter and jelly
Coconut layer cake
Large glass milk and cream mixed
Coffee or tea, cream and sugar

Bedtime

Sandwich: 2 slices bread, 2 ounces meat or substitute (*See* page 148), butter and/or mayonnaise
Large glass milk and cream mixed

REDUCTION DIETS

The following are general rules to be observed with a reduction diet:

1. No sugar is to be used. Saccharine or Cyclamate-free sweetener may be used instead.

2. Fruits should be fresh only, or canned without sugar (water pack).
3. Clear coffee or tea or unsweetened lemonade is allowed between meals.
4. Meats should be lean and prepared without the addition of fat (broiled, boiled or baked).
5. No salad dressings are allowed unless substituted for the butter allowance.
6. A small serving of potato, corn or lima beans may be substituted for a slice of bread.
7. Fat-free broth may be taken as desired unless salt is restricted.
8. A satisfactory weight reduction is 8-10 pounds per month.

It is not abnormal for weight to remain stationary for the first three or four weeks while on a reduction diet. Do not become discouraged. With perseverance a weight loss will eventually follow.

DIET III

APPROXIMATELY 1,400 CALORIES
WITH 85 GRAMS PROTEIN

The average individual should be able to lose weight satisfactorily on this plan, unless confined to bed.

MEAL PLAN

Breakfast

Small glass fruit juice (4 ounces) or unsweetened fruit
1 egg—not fried
1 slice toast
1 pat butter or margarine
Large glass skim milk (8 ounces)
Clear coffee or tea

Lunch

Sandwich: 2 slices bread, 2 ounces meat or substitute (*See* page 148),
    1 pat butter or mayonnaise, lettuce
Raw vegetable salad
1 serving fresh or unsweetened fruit
Clear coffee or tea

Dinner

5 ounces meat or substitute (*See* page 148)
1 small serving potato (boiled, baked, or mashed only), corn or lima
   beans
Cooked vegetable
Raw vegetable salad
1 slice bread with 1 pat butter
1 serving fresh or unsweetened fruit
Large glass skim milk (8 ounces)
Clear coffee or tea

SAMPLE MENUS OF DIET III

Choice No. 1

Breakfast

Sliced orange
Poached egg
1 slice toast with 1 pat butter
Large glass skim milk
Clear coffee or tea

Lunch

Sandwich: 2 slices bread, 2 slices cheese, butter or mayonnaise,
   lettuce
Celery sticks
Fresh pineapple without sugar
Clear coffee or tea

Dinner

2 broiled lamb chops
Small boiled potato
Vinegar beets
Sliced tomato salad with ½ cup cottage cheese
1 slice bread with 1 pat butter
Cantaloupe (¼ of one medium-sized)
Large glass skim milk
Clear coffee or tea

Choice No. 2

Breakfast

Small glass grapefruit juice
Soft-cooked egg
1 slice toast with 1 pat butter
Large glass skim milk
Clear coffee or tea

Lunch

1 frankfurter bun
2 frankfurters
Catsup, mustard
Head lettuce wedge and mayonnaise
Small apple
Clear coffee or tea

Dinner

Broiled ground beef patties (5 ounces)
Corn
Asparagus
Carrot curls
1 slice bread with 1 pat buter
Small fresh pear
Large glass skim milk
Clear coffee or tea

DIET IV

APPROXIMATELY 1,000 CALORIES
WITH 80 GRAMS PROTEIN

MEAL PLAN

Breakfast

Small glass of fruit juice or 1 serving fresh or unsweetened fruit
One egg not fried
1 slice dry toast
Small glass skim milk (4 ounces)
Clear coffee or tea

Lunch

Sandwich: 2 slices bread, 2 ounces meat or substitute (*See* page 148),
    no butter or mayonnaise, lettuce
Raw vegetables if desired
1 serving fresh or unsweetened canned fruit
Small glass skim milk (4 ounces)
Clear coffee or tea

Dinner

5 ounces meat or substitute (*See* page 148)
Cooked vegetable
Salad (Vegetable)
1 serving fresh or unsweetened canned fruit
1 large glass skim milk (8 ounces) or fat-free buttermilk
Clear coffee or tea

SAMPLE MENUS OF DIET IV

Choice No. 1

Breakfast

Small glass orange juice
1 poached egg on 1 slice dry toast
Small glass skim milk
Clear coffee or tea

Lunch

Sandwich: 2 slices bread, 2 slices cheese, lettuce, pickles
Tossed vegetable salad with vinegar or lemon juice
Small apple
Small glass skim milk
Clear coffee or tea

Dinner

Broiled chicken—1 leg and 1 breast (small)
Asparagus
Head lettuce salad with lemon juice
Fresh grapes
Large glass skim milk
Clear coffee or tea

Choice No. 2

Breakfast

½ grapefruit
1 soft-cooked egg
1 slice dry toast
Small glass skim milk
Clear coffee or tea

Lunch

Sandwich: 2 slices bread, 2 slices roast beef, lettuce, pickles
Celery hearts, radishes
½ banana
Small glass skim milk
Clear coffee or tea

Dinner

Two large broiled veal chops
Green beans
Coleslaw with vinegar
1 orange
Large glass skim milk
Clear coffee or tea

LOW-SODIUM DIETS

The following diet is suitable for an individual of normal weight who must restrict his sodium intake. Such restriction must be carried out only under the direction of a physician.

DIET V

600 mg SODIUM DIET

Special Instructions:

1. Do not use salt in cooking or on food afterwards.
2. Read the labels on canned foods. Do not use food labeled as containing salt or sodium.
3. Do not use soda, salt or baking powder in cooking or as a medication.

CHECK LIST OF FOODS FOR LOW SODIUM DIET

BEVERAGES

List A, Allowed
Tea, coffee, 1 pint milk per day to be used as beverage or in cooking, fruit juices, salt-free tomato juice, Coca-Cola, ginger ale, root beer, special dietetic soft drinks low in sodium

List B Avoid
Vegetable juices, Dutch process cocoa

BREADS AND BREADSTUFFS

Salt-free bread, Salt-free Melba toast

Crackers, hot breads, breads containing salt

CEREALS

Salt-free cooked cereal as oatmeal, Cream of Wheat, corn meal, Wheatena, Ralston, dry Puffed Wheat, Puffed Rice, shredded wheat

Cereals cooked with salt, enriched cereals (may use unenriched), dry cereals not listed

DAIRY PRODUCTS

Cream
Eggs—1 daily, cooked any way; use unsalted butter or unsalted cooking fat. More than one a day may be used if substituted for meat

Cheeses
Salted butter, oleomargarine

DESSERTS

Fruit, gelatin desserts, fruit ice. Milk puddings and ice cream may be substituted for milk allowance. Pies made without salt

All bakery products made with soda, salt or baking powder. Commercial ready-made mixes (cakes, cookies, gelatin such as Jello)

FRUITS

Any, cooked or raw

MEATS

Beef, lamb, veal, poultry, fresh fish (except shellfish), unsalted canned tuna and salmon, fresh pork, liver

All smoked, preserved, canned meats, ham, bacon, luncheon meats, frankfurters, sausage, corned beef, chipped beef, kidneys, frozen fish, shellfish, canned, salted or smoked fish

VEGETABLES

Fresh or frozen vegetables except those listed to avoid. Canned vegetables specially prepared without salt (except those listed). Onions, Brussels sprouts, broccoli, cauliflower, cabbage, green pepper, navy and lima beans, kidney beans and turnips, unless they cause gas

Canned vegetables, fresh or frozen spinach, beets, beet greens, kale or other dark green vegetables, celery, frozen peas and lima beans

Potato or Substitute
White or sweet potato, rice, spaghetti, noodles, macaroni, hominy grits

Potato chips

MISCELLANEOUS

Seasoning
All seasonings except those listed to avoid.

Salt, prepared seasoning salts (onion, garlic, or celery salts)

Salad Dressings
Salad oil made without salt; vinegar or lemon juice

Commercial salad dressings

Soups
Clear soups with allowed vegetables. Cream soups if substituted for milk allowed

Canned soups, bouillon cubes

Sweets
Jelly, preserves, jams, honey, sugar, plain hard candies, unsweetened chocolate

Molasses, chocolate candy bars, brown sugar

MEAL PLAN

Breakfast

Fruit or juice
Salt-free cereal
1 egg
Salt-free toast
Sweet butter
Milk as allowed
Coffee
Sugar

Lunch

Meat, fish, chicken
Potato or substitute
Vegetable as allowed
Salad if desired
Salt-free bread
Sweet butter
Fruit or dessert as allowed
Coffee, tea, or milk as allowed

Dinner

Meat, fish, chicken
Potato or substitute
Vegetable as allowed
Salad if desired
Salt-free bread
Sweet butter
Fruit or dessert as allowed
Coffee, tea or milk as allowed

When weight reduction must be combined with a low-sodium diet, refer to Diet V for general principles of the sodium-restricted diet. In addition, the following modifications must be observed to reduce the caloric intake.

1. Use fresh or unsweetened fruit and juices only as desserts.
2. Meats should be lean and prepared without the addition of fat (baking, broiling or boiling).

3. Use only unsalted bread and butter.
4. Use no sugar, soft drinks or preserves, jellies, honey, etc.
5. Omit celery, spinach and other dark greens, beets and frozen lima beans and peas.
6. Use no meat broths or meat extracts.
7. Eat only the foods listed below.

REDUCTION DIET VI-A

APPROXIMATELY 1,100 CALORIES WITH 65 GRAMS PROTEIN AND 200-300 mg SODIUM
(Using a low-sodium milk such as Lonalac
by Mead-Johnson)

MEAL PLAN

Breakfast

Small glass fruit juice or unsweetened fruit
1 egg (not fried)
1 slice dry, unsalted toast
1 glass (8 ounces) low-sodium milk
Clear coffee or tea

Lunch

2 ounces unsalted meat (*See* page 163)
½ slice unsalted bread (no butter)
Raw vegetables if desired
1 serving fresh or unsweetened canned fruit
Small glass low sodium milk (4 ounces)
Clear coffee or tea

Dinner

3 ounces unsalted meat (*See* page 163)
Cooked vegetable (no potato, corn or lima beans)
Raw vegetable salad
½ slice unsalted bread (no butter)
1 serving fresh or unsweetened canned fruit
Small glass low sodium milk (4 ounces)
Clear coffee or tea

The following supply 2 ounces of unsalted meat or its equivalent:
A) ½ cup unsalted (dietetic pack) salmon or tuna
B) 4 tablespoons unsalted peanut butter
C) 1 medium slice of any fresh meat (beef, lamb, veal, poultry or *lean* fresh pork)
D) ½ cup dry cottage cheese

The following supply 3 ounces of unsalted meat or its equivalent:
A) 3 ounces fresh fish (except shellfish)
B) 1 large veal or lean pork loin chop
C) 2 large lamb chops
D) 1 slice, approximately 4″ x 2″ x ½″ of any fresh meat, such as a roast, steak, or fowl

The following supply 5 ounces of unsalted meat or its equivalent:
A) 5 ounces fresh fish (except shellfish)
B) 2 large veal or pork loin chops
C) 3 large lamb chops
D) 2 slices, each 4″ x 2½″ x ½″, of a fresh meat—roast, steak or fowl, etc.
E) 1 leg and 1 breast chicken

SAMPLE MENU OF REDUCTION DIET VI-A

Breakfast

½ grapefruit
Poached egg on 1 slice dry, unsalted toast
8-ounce glass low-sodium milk
Clear coffee or tea

Lunch

Cold plate:
    ½ cup unsalted salmon with vinegar
    ½ slice unsalted bread
    sliced-tomato-and-lettuce salad
Small apple
Small glass low-sodium milk (4 ounces)
Clear coffee or tea

Dinner

3 ounces unsalted pot roast of beef
Carrots
Head lettuce salad with mixed vinegar and saccharine
½ slice unsalted bread
Sliced orange
Small glass low-sodium milk (4 ounces)
Clear coffee or tea

REDUCTION DIET VI-B

APPROXIMATELY 1,000 CALORIES WITH 60 GRAMS PROTEIN AND 300 mg SODIUM
(Without the use of a low-sodium milk;
calcium tablets may be indicated)

MEAL PLAN

Breakfast

1 serving unsweetened fruit juice or fruit
2 eggs, not fried
1 slice unsalted toast
1 pat unsalted butter
Clear coffee or tea

Lunch

Sandwich: 2 slices unsalted bread, 2 ounces unsalted meat or substitute (*See* page 163), lettuce
Raw vegetable if desired
1 serving fresh or unsweetened canned fruit
Clear coffee or tea

Dinner

3 ounces unsalted meat (*See* page 163)
Unsalted cooked vegetable
Raw vegetable salad
1 slice unsalted bread
1 pat unsalted butter
1 serving fresh or unsweetened canned fruit
Clear coffee or tea

SAMPLE MENU OF DIET VI-B

Breakfast

Small glass orange juice
2 soft-cooked eggs
1 slice unsalted toast
1 pat unsalted butter
Clear coffee or tea

Lunch

Sandwich: 2 slices unsalted bread, 4 tablespoons unsalted peanut
butter, lettuce
Fresh pineapple without sugar
Clear coffee or tea

Dinner

3 ounces unsalted broiled liver
Unsalted asparagus
Tossed vegetable salad with lemon juice
1 slice unsalted bread
1 pat unsalted butter
Fresh plum
Clear coffee or tea
A small serving of corn, potato or canned lima beans may be sub-
stituted for the bread.

DIET VII—*Gout*

Patients with gout must avoid foods containing substances that help produce uric acid. These are found primarily in meats, whole-grain cereals and a few vegetables. In addition, fats and alcoholic beverages are taboo; the former because they interfere with the body's elimination of uric acid; the latter because they bring on acute attacks. On the following pages there will be found a check list of foods telling which to eat and which to avoid, and then detailed menus for a gouty patient of normal weight (2,000 calories), and a gouty patient who must reduce (1,200 calories).

CHECK LIST OF FOODS FOR GOUTY PATIENTS:

List A Always avoid	List B Eat sparingly	List C Eat as desired
BEVERAGES		
Alcohol in any form		Buttermilk
		Carbonated drinks
		Chocolate
		Cocoa
		Coffee
		Milk
		Postum
		Sanka
		Tea
		Fruit Juices
BREADS and BREADSTUFFS		
	Pumpernickel	Cornbread
	Whole wheat	French bread
	Graham bread	White bread
	Graham crackers	Soda crackers
		Crackers, cookies and cakes, unless made from whole-wheat, oat or rye flour

CEREALS

Whole-grain cereals	Cornflakes
Shredded wheat	Cream of Wheat
Whole bran	Farina
Puffed wheat	Post Toasties
	Puffed rice
	Rice flakes
	Rice Krispies
	White corn meal

DAIRY PRODUCTS

Butter	Buttermilk
Oleomargarine	Cheese
	Eggs
	Milk

List A	*List B*	*List C*
Always avoid	*Eat sparingly*	*Eat as desired*

DESSERTS

Ice cream	Blancmange
Pastries	Cake
Pie	Gelatin
	Jello
	Puddings
	Bread
	Butterscotch
	Chocolate
	Rice
	Tapioca

MEATS

Anchovies	Bacon
Brains	Beef
Clams	Bologna
Duck	Chicken
Goose	Crabmeat
Kidneys	Fish (other than those
Liver	listed)
Meat extracts	Frankfurters
Pheasant	Frogs' legs

Pigeon
Pork
Rabbit
Sausage (pork)
Scallops
Scrapple
Shellfish
Shrimp
Squab
Sweetbreads
Tongue

Ham
Herring
Lamb
Salmon
Tuna
Turkey

VEGETABLES

List A *Always avoid*	*List B* *Eat sparingly*	*List C* *Eat as desired*	
	Asparagus	Artichokes	Parsnips
	Beans	Beets	Potatoes
	Kidney	Broccoli	Sweet
	Lima	Brussels	White
	Navy	sprouts	Pumpkin
	Cauliflower	Cabbage	Radishes
	Mushrooms	Carrots	Rice
	Onions	Celery	Rutabagas
	Peas	Corn	Sauerkraut
	Spinach	Cucumbers	Spaghetti
		Eggplant	String beans
		Endive	Squash
		Hominy	Swiss chard
		Lettuce	Tomatoes
		Macaroni	Turnips
		Noodles	
		Okra	

MISCELLANEOUS

Gravies	Nuts	Candy
Meat soups	Bouillon	Condiments
	Cream soups	Fruits of all kinds
	Peanut butter	Soups (except
	Mayonnaise	bouillon)
	French dressing	Tapioca
	Russian dressing	Vinegar

SAMPLE MENUS OF DIET VII: 2,000 CALORIES

SUNDAY	MONDAY	TUESDAY

Breakfast

SUNDAY	MONDAY	TUESDAY
Orange juice—½ cup	½ grapefruit	Sliced banana
Farina—½ cup	Farina—½ cup	Soft-cooked egg
Poached egg	Coddled egg	Cornflakes with cream
Toast—1 slice	Toast—1 slice	(¼ cup)
Butter—1 tsp.	Butter—1 tsp.	Toast—1 slice
Cream—¼ cup	Coffee	Butter—1 tsp.
Coffee	Cream—¼ cup	Coffee

Lunch

SUNDAY	MONDAY	TUESDAY
Broiled chicken—¼ chicken	Macaroni & cheese (½ c. macaroni, 2 slices cheese & ½ cup milk)	American cheese—2 slices
Buttered corn—½ cup	Buttered beets	Brussels sprouts
Green beans—½ cup	Tossed green salad with lemon	Steamed rice
Tomato salad	Bread—1 slice	Celery sticks
Roll—1	Butter—1 tsp.	Saltines—5
Butter—1 tsp.	Fruit cocktail—½ cup	Tapioca—½ cup
Fruit Jello	Milk—1 cup	Milk—1 cup

Dinner

SUNDAY	MONDAY	TUESDAY
Cottage cheese—3 oz.	Cream of mushroom soup—1 cup	Broiled steak
Buttered carrots—½ cup	Tomato stuffed with cottage cheese—mayonnaise (1 tsp.)	Mashed potatoes
Baked potato (small)	Broccoli	Carrots
Lettuce wedge—lemon	Boiled potato	1 slice French bread
Saltines—5	Hard roll	Tomato salad
Butter—1 tsp.	Butter—1 tsp.	Milk—1 cup
Custard—½ cup	Rice pudding—½ cup	Peaches—2 halves
Milk—1 cup	Milk	
	Coffee	
	Cream—1 tsp.	

WEDNESDAY	THURSDAY	FRIDAY

Breakfast

Tomato juice	Applesauce—1 cup	Orange
Egg—1	Farina—½ cup	Milk toast—1 cup milk
Rice Krispies	Fried egg	(1 slice toast, 1 tsp.
Toast—1 slice	Toast—1 slice	butter, 1 tsp. sugar)
Butter—1 tsp.	Butter—1 tsp.	1 scrambled egg
Cream—¼ cup	Cream—¼ cup	Coffee
Coffee	Sugar—1 tsp.	Cream—1 tsp.

Lunch

Ham—3 oz.	American cheese—	Broiled crab cake (2
Buttered potatoes	2 slices	small)
String beans	Corn O'Brien	Buttered cabbage—1
Sliced cucumber/	Buttered beets	cup
lemon juice	Pear salad	Carrot sticks—radishes
1 Corn muffin	Bread—1 slice	Hard roll—1
Butter—1 tsp.	Butter—1 tsp.	Butter—1 tsp.
Pineapple—2 slices	Baked custard	Fresh fruit cup
Milk—1 cup	Milk—1 cup	Milk—1 cup

Dinner

Omelet—3 eggs	Roast beef—3 oz.	2 poached eggs on
Baked potato with	Baked potato	rusk
butter	Buttered onions	Stewed tomatoes
Cauliflower	Tomato salad with	Baked Hubbard
Tossed green salad	1 tsp. mayonnaise	Squash
with lemon	Roll—1	Pear salad with 1 tsp.
White bread—1 slice	Butter—1 tsp.	cream cheese
Butter—1 tsp.	Fresh fruit cup	Plain Jello—½ cup
Vanilla pudding	Milk—1 cup	Milk—1 cup

SATURDAY	SUNDAY	MONDAY

Breakfast

Grapefruit juice—½	Tomato juice	Strawberries—1 cup
cup	French toast—2	Farina—½ cup
Poached egg—1	slices, 2 tsp. syrup	Egg—poached—1
Cornflakes—¾ cup	Coffee	Toast—1 slice

Breakfast

Toast—1 slice
Butter—1 tsp.
Cream—¼ cup
Sugar—2 tsp.
Coffee

Milk—2 tsp.

Butter—1 tsp.
Cream—¼ cup
Coffee

Lunch

Tomato wedge with
  tuna salad—½ cup
Buttered potato (1
  small)
Broccoli—aver. serv.
Saltines—5
Sweet peaches—2
  halves
Milk—1 cup

Sliced turkey
Baked potato
Green beans
Pepper rings—radishes
  —celery
Roll—1
Butter—1 tsp.
Ice cream—½ cup
Milk—1 cup

Cream of tomato
  soup
Baked potato—
  glazed carrot
Peach & cottage
  cheese (3 tsp.)
  salad
Saltines—5
Butter—1 tsp.
Custard—½ cup
Milk—1 cup

Dinner

Hamburger pattie—
  3 oz.
Rutabagas—½ cup
Green beans—½ cup
Tossed green salad
  —1 tsp. mayon-
  naise
Fresh apple
Milk—1 cup

Creamed eggs/toast
Broiled tomatoes
Broccoli
Lettuce wedge—
  mayonnaise
Sliced pineapple—2
  slices
Milk—1 cup

Cream of potato
  soup
Egg à la goldenrod
Buttered parsnips
Green salad with 1
  slice of cheese
Baked apple

TUESDAY	WEDNESDAY	THURSDAY

Breakfast

Banana—1
Puffed rice
Egg—fried in 1 tsp.
  butter
Toast—1 slice
Butter—1 tsp.

Blended juice—½
  cup
Poached egg—1
Toast—2 slices
Milk—1 cup
Coffee

Pineapple juice—½
  cup
Rice Krispies
Soft-cooked egg—1
Toast—1 slice
Butter—1 tsp.

Breakfast

Milk—½ cup
Cream—¼ cup
Coffee
Sugar—2 tsp.

Sugar—2 tsp.

Cream—¼ cup
Coffee
Sugar—2 tsp.

Lunch

American cheese
 (2 slices) sandwich
Potato chips
Tomato salad
Mayonnaise—1 tsp.
Tapioca—½ cup
Milk—1 cup

Vegetable soup
 (seasoned with 1
 tsp. butter)
Cottage cheese—½
 cup with tomato
 wedge
Saltines—5
Milk—1 cup
Vanilla ice cream—
 ½ cup

Egg salad—(2 eggs)
 sandwich—2 slices
Potato chips
Celery sticks
Milk—1 cup
Fruit Jello

Dinner

Steak—3 oz.
Mashed potatoes—
 ½ cup
Buttered broccoli
Lettuce wedge with
 French dressing
Roll—1
Butter—1 tsp.
Loaf cake—1 slice
 (small)
Milk—1 cup

Veal chops—2
Beets—½ cup
Cauliflower—average
 serving
Corn muffin—2
Butter—2 tsp.
Milk—1 cup
½ grapefruit

Salisbury steak
Glazed carrots—½
 cup
Broiled onions
Green salad with 1
 tsp. mayonnaise
Milk—1 cup
Peaches—2 halves

FRIDAY   **SATURDAY**

Breakfast

Orange juice—½
 cup
Farina—½ cup
Scrambled egg—1
Toast—1 slice
Butter—1 tsp.
Cream—¼ cup
Coffee
Sugar—1 tsp.

Applesause—1 cup
Cornflakes—¾ cup
Poached egg
Toast—1 slice
Butter—1 tsp.
Cream—¼ cup
Coffee

Lunch

Cottage cheese—3 oz. with 2 slices of pineapple
Potato chips—1 cup
Saltines—5
Butter—2 tsp.
Milk—1 cup
Rice pudding—½ cup

Omelet—3 eggs
Broiled tomatoes
Carrots—½ cup
Toast—2 slices
Butter—2 tsp.
Jelly—1 tsp.
Milk—1 cup
Orange—1

Dinner

Egg soufflé—3 eggs
Baked potato—1
Summer squash—½ cup
Tomato juice—1 cup
Milk—1 cup
Roll—1
Butter—2 tsp.
Sweet pears—2 halves

Roast beef—3 oz.
Brussels sprouts—6
Beets—½ cup
Coleslaw—½ cup
Corn muffin—2
Milk—1 cup
½ grapefruit

SAMPLE MENU DIET VIIA: 1,200 CALORIES

SUNDAY	MONDAY	TUESDAY

Breakfast

Orange juice—½ cup	Grapefruit—½	Sliced banana—½
Poached egg—1	Coddled egg—1	Soft-cooked egg—1
Toast—1 slice	Toast—1 slice	Toast—1 slice
Butter—1 tsp.	Butter—1 tsp.	Butter—1 tsp.
Milk—½ cup	Milk—½ cup	Milk—½ cup
Coffee	Coffee	Coffee
Saccharin (if desired)	Saccharin (if desired)	Saccharin(if desired)

Lunch

Broiled chicken—¼ chicken	American cheese—2 slices	Hard-boiled egg—2
Green beans—½ cup	Beets—½ cup	Brussels sprouts—6
Tomato salad	Tossed salad with lemon	Celery sticks
Roll—1		Saltines—5
		Grapes—10

Lunch

Butter—1 tsp.	Bread—1 slice	Milk—1 cup
Unsweetened pears —2 halves	Butter—1 tsp.	
Milk—1 cup	Unsweetened fruit cocktail—½ cup	
	Milk—1 cup	

Dinner

Cottage cheese—3 oz.	Tomato stuffed with cottage cheese	Broiled steak—3 oz.
Carrots—½ cup		Carrots—½ cup
Lettuce wedge with lemon	Broccoli—average serving	Tomato salad
Saltines—5	Hard roll—1	French bread—1 slice
Fresh apple—1	Orange sections—½ cup	Unsweetened peaches —2 halves
Milk—1 cup	Milk—1 cup	Milk—1 cup

WEDNESDAY	THURSDAY	FRIDAY

Breakfast

Tomato juice—1 cup	Unsweetened apple-sauce—½ cup	Orange juice—½ cup
Egg—poached—1	Soft-cooked egg—1	Coddled egg—1
Toast—1 slice	Toast—1 slice	Toast—1 slice
Butter—1 tsp.	Butter—1 tsp.	Butter—1 tsp.
Milk—½ cup	Milk—½ cup	Milk—½ cup
Coffee	Coffee	Coffee
Saccharin (if desired)	Saccharin (if desired)	Saccharin (if desired)

Lunch

Ham—3 oz.	Salmon salad—½ cup with tomato wedge	Broiled crab cake—1
String beans—½ cup		Boiled cabbage—1 cup
Sliced cucumber—lemon juice	Carrot—celery sticks	
Corn muffin—1	Bread—1 slice	Carrot sticks—radishes
Butter—1 tsp.	Grapes—10	Hard roll—1
Unsweetened pine-apple—2 slices	Milk—1 cup	Butter—1 tsp.
Milk—1 cup		Fresh fruit cup—½ cup
		Milk—1 cup

Dinner

Omelet–2 eggs	Roast beef–3 oz.	2 poached eggs on rusk
Cauliflower–1 cup	Baked potato–1 small	
Tossed green salad with lemon	Boiled onions–3 small	Stewed tomatoes–1 cup
Bread–1 slice	Butter–1 tsp.	Baked Hubbard squash–1 cup
Fresh orange–1	Unsweetened fruit cocktail–½ cup	Unsweetened pears –2 halves
	Milk–1 cup	Milk–1 cup

SATURDAY	SUNDAY	MONDAY

Breakfast

Grapefruit juice–½ cup	Tomato juice–1 cup	Grapefruit–½
Poached egg–1	Soft-cooked egg–1	Scrambled egg–1
Toast–1 slice	Toast–1 slice	Toast–1 slice
Butter–1 tsp.	Butter–1 tsp.	Milk–½ cup
Milk–½ cup	Milk–½ cup	Coffee
Coffee	Coffee	Saccharin (if desired)
Saccharin (if desired)	Saccharin (if desired)	

Lunch

Tomato wedge with cottage cheese–½ cup	Sliced turkey–3 oz.	Cottage cheese–3 oz. with unsweetened pears–2 halves and lettuce
Broccoli–aver. serv.	Baked potato–1 small	
Saltines–5	Green beans–½ cup	Tomato juice–1 cup
Unsweetened peaches –2 halves	Pepper rings–radishes–celery	Saltines–5
Milk–1 cup	Butter–1 tsp.	Milk–1 cup
	Baked apple–no sugar	
	Milk–1 cup	

Dinner

Hamburger patties –3 oz.	2 scrambled eggs	Lamb chops–2
Roll–1	Broiled tomato	Rice–½ cup
Raw onion–½	Lettuce wedge with lemon	Carrots–½ cup
Tomato salad	Toast–1 slice	Green salad with lemon

Dinner

Fresh apple—1	Unsweetened pine-	Butter—1 tsp.
Milk—1 cup	apple—2 slices	Grapes—10
	Milk—1 cup	Milk—1 cup

TUESDAY	WEDNESDAY	THURSDAY

Breakfast

Banana—1	Blended juice—½	Unsweetened pine-
Cornflakes—1 cup	cup	apple juice—⅓ cup
Milk—½ cup	Poached egg—1	Soft-cooked egg—1
Coffee	Toast—1 slice	Toast—1 slice
Saccharin (if desired)	Butter—1 tsp.	Butter—1 tsp.
	Milk—½ cup	Milk—½ cup
	Coffee	Coffee
	Saccharin (if desired)	Saccharin (if desired)

Lunch

American cheese (2 slices) sandwich	Cottage cheese (cup) salad with tomato wedge	Egg salad—(1 egg) sandwich
Tomato salad	Saltines—5	Radishes—celery
Milk—1 cup	Milk—1 cup	Milk—1 cup
Fresh apple	Unsweetened fruit cocktail—½ cup	Banana—½

Dinner

Steak—3 oz.	Veal chop—1 large	Hamburger pattie —3 oz.
Mashed potatoes— ½ cup	Beets—½ cup	Carrots—½ cup
Broccoli—average serving	Cauliflower—½ cup	Boiled onions—3 small
	Corn muffin—1	
Lettuce with lemon	Butter—1 tsp.	Green salad with lemon
Milk—1 cup	Milk—1 cup	Milk—1 cup
Fresh orange—1	½ grapefruit	Unsweetened peaches —2 halves

FRIDAY	SATURDAY

Breakfast

Orange juice—½ cup	Unsweetened apple-
Rice Krispies—1 cup	sauce—½ cup
Milk—½ cup	Poached egg—1
Coffee	Toast—1 slice
Saccharin (if desired)	Butter—1 tsp.
	Coffee
	Saccharin (if desired)

Lunch

Cottage cheese (3 oz.) with pineapple (2 slices)	Omelet—2 eggs
Corn muffin—1	Broiled tomato
Butter—1 tsp.	Toast—1 slice
Milk—1 cup	Jelly—1 tsp.
	Milk—1 cup
	Orange—1

Dinner

Lamb—3 oz.	Roast beef—3 oz.
Baked potato—1	Brussels sprouts—6
Summer squash—1 cup	Beets—½ cup
Tomato juice—1 cup	Coleslaw—½ cup
Milk—1 cup	Milk—1 cup
Unsweetened pears —2 halves	Grapefruit—½

Appendix B: Exercises

On the following pages will be found exercises to help over-come stiffness and increase motion in the joints. Postural exercises designed to help you stand and walk correctly are also included. The exact time spent exercising will depend on many factors—your age, general health, severity of your arthritis. Never attempt to do all the exercises listed at one time. In general, they are ar-ranged in order of difficulty. You should do the first two or three exercises several times a day for several days—and then proceed to others, increasing the time from an initial period of five min-utes to about twenty minutes. They should be done in a well-ventilated room of proper temperature (about 70°). Prior to the exercise period, heat should be applied as described in the section titled "Local Applications of Heat" in Chapter IX. You will note that, in general, exercises for the extremities are described for both sides of the body. Many times, only one shoulder or one hip is affected. In such cases, the exercises are to be modified as necessary to fit the particular situation. Here, as in other parts of this manual, you must work in close cooperation with your phy-sician. The following rules should always be observed.

RULES FOR LOCAL EXERCISES

1. Never over-exert or do the exercises too strenuously; do them slowly, rhythmically and carefully. Exercise until you just begin to feel tired—stop before you become fatigued.

2. Do not slight the exercises by doing them halfway. An exercise should be done to the fullest degree or not at all. If a joint is taken through only part of its possible range of motion, the value of the exercise is lost.

3. If a joint is acutely inflamed, put it through complete range of motion very gently to maintain the range. Do not force heavy exercises during a flare-up. This may cause the inflammation to become worse. When not exercising, always maintain the joint in a good postural position.

4. Never allow the part to be pulled, jerked or handled roughly.

5. Exaggeration of pain in the joint, persisting for more than one hour after the exercises have been performed, indicates that they have been too strenuous. They should be less vigorous at the next session.

6. Following an exercise program, lie down and rest for one hour. It is not necessary that you sleep, but you must relax completely (eyes closed and not listening to radio or television).

7. Take five slow deep breaths at the start, at the finish, and several times during each exercise period.

RULES OF POSTURE

Maintaining correct posture is one of the most important therapeutic measure in any rheumatic disease. It is so easy when one has pain, to slump and slouch, and to hold the hands or legs in twisted positions. Yet this may bring about irreversible damage. Muscles may become tightened, holding the spine bent forward—or a joint in a deformed position. Such deformities may take months to correct—so an ounce of prevention is worth a pound of cure. The maintenance of proper posture permits the blood to circulate through all muscles and joints and so assist nature in the healing processes. The following exercises are, therefore, important to all readers of this book. There is nothing mysterious or complicated about them. Indeed, many are the simple "setting-up" exercises taught in high school gym classes or army training camps. The important thing is to do some of them regularly every day.

Correct Standing Position: Stand erect with the body held as tall as possible without strain, chin horizontal (back and in, not tilting), chest forward and up, abdominal and gluteal (buttock) muscles tightened, feet six inches apart with weight on the front and outer borders of the feet, toes pointing out at 5°.

Correct Walking: Start with the toes pointing out about five degrees with correct standing posture. Place one foot forward and strike that heel to the floor, roll on the outside of the foot to the ball, roll in on the ball of that foot and push off from the great toe while bringing the opposite foot forward to heel strike on that side.

Walk at a natural, even gait. Raise the feet high enough from the floor to avoid shuffling. Keep the body erect and do not waddle or sway.

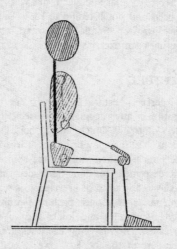

DIAGRAM 1

Correct Sitting Position: (Diagrams 1 & 2): Sit erect with body held tall and well back in chair, weight on hips, not spine. Do not slouch. Keep abdominal muscles tightened, and chest forward and up. In leaning forward while sitting, bend forward

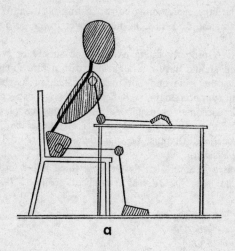

a

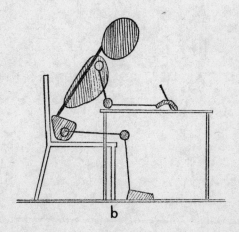

b

DIAGRAM 2

only at the hips, maintaining correct sitting position. When looking down at the desk flex the neck—never lower portions of the
spine.

Shoes: A properly fitting oxford shoe should be worn at all
times. This should have a straight last with a firm inner counter.
Heels must be wide and not over one inch in height. Certain
additional supports may be indicated. Sponge rubber supports
for the longitudinal or metatarsal arches may be placed inside
the shoe. Externally, a special heel, a metatarsal bar or wedge
may be needed. All must be individually prescribed by the attending physician.

Exercises in several of the groups which follow are listed as
being done from the "dorsal recumbent position." This means

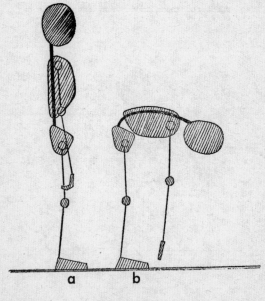

Diagram 3

lying flat on the back, face up, legs extended, arms at the sides. Generally a pillow is not used under the head. The "prone position" means lying on the abdomen and chest, face down or turned partially to one side to permit breathing.

POSTURAL EXERCISES
FOR THE BACK AND HIPS

Assume Correct Standing Position

1. DIAGRAM 3: Bend the trunk evenly, bending the entire spine as far as possible and attempt to touch the toes with the finger tips keeping the knees straight and the head down; do not force. Hold for count of two and return.

2. DIAGRAM 4: Clasp hands behind hips. Bend forward

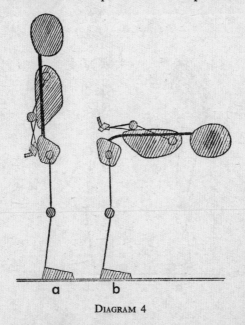

a   b

DIAGRAM 4

only at hips, keeping rest of spine rigid and bringing body to a right angle. Hold for count of two and return.

3. DIAGRAM 5: Stand four inches away from the wall, back toward the wall. Bend body forward at the hips until back is arched and buttocks touch the wall; slowly straighten up until the lower back, shoulders, and head touch the wall. Try to flatten the entire spine against the wall. Hold for a count of five and relax. Then try to straighten up the whole spine away from the wall.

4. Raise the right leg, bring the knee to the chest; clasp

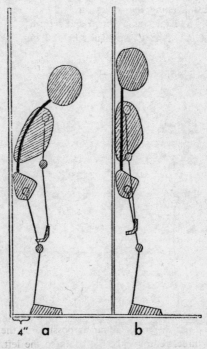

4"   a   b

DIAGRAM 5

it tightly with both hands, and tighten abdomen. Hold for count of five. Lower right leg and repeat with the left. If balance is poor stand with side next to the wall.

5. Move right leg backward as far as possible keeping knees straight and toes pointing straight ahead. Hold for count of two and return. Repeat same with left leg.

6. Move right leg out to side as far as possible, keeping knee straight and toes pointing straight ahead. Hold for count of two and return. Repeat same with left leg.

7. Place right hand on hip and left hand over head. Bend to the right as far as possible. Hold for the count of two and return. Repeat, placing left hand on hip and right hand over head, bending to the left.

8. Place arms out to side at shoulder level. Move hands backward as far as possible. Hold for count of five. Return to starting position.

9. Tighten abdominal muscles. Hold for the count of ten and relax.

10. Place hands on lower ribs, thumbs toward the rear, fingers toward the front, tighten abdominal muscles, now inhale deeply, elevating chest and expanding lower ribs. Hold for count of three, exhale slowly keeping chest elevated, then relax.

Assume and Hold Erect Sitting Position on Floor

11. Spread legs apart, turn toes in (pigeon toe) and raise arms to the sides shoulder high. Now, rotate body and swing right hand to left foot, left arm to rear. Hold for the count of two and return. Repeat with left hand to the right foot.

12. Spread legs wide apart, grasp ankles and pull head and trunk toward floor between the legs. Hold for the count of two and return.

13. Sit with hands at back of neck, chest high, elbows well back. Slowly twist the trunk as far as possible to the right. Hold for count of three, return and twist trunk to the left.

14. Resting arms on the floor in back, lift the right leg knee

straight, six inches off the floor. Hold for the count of five and
return. Repeat lifting the left leg.

15. Sit with legs straight and together, hands at back of
neck; bring right knee up to chest with foot off the floor without
changing position of the trunk. Hold for the count of two and
return. Repeat with the left knee.

Dorsal Recumbent Position

(Lie on Back, Face Upward)

16. DIAGRAM 6: Bend the knees and place the feet on
the floor. Inhale deeply and flatten the back against the floor by
tipping the hips, tightening the abdominal and gluteal (buttock)
muscles. Hold for the count of five, exhale and return by re-
laxing muscles. Raising the head a few inches from the floor
will help maintain the back flat against the floor.

17. Place the hands under the neck with the arms touching
the floor. Keep the head on floor and raise the chest, arching
the upper back as much as possible. Hold for the count of three
and lower the chest.

18. Place arms over head, palm up. Slowly swing arms upward and forward, raising first the head and then the chest while
rounding the back and keeping the knees straight. Continue in

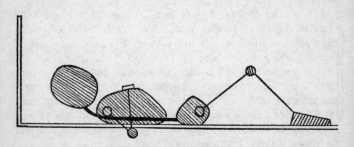

DIAGRAM 6

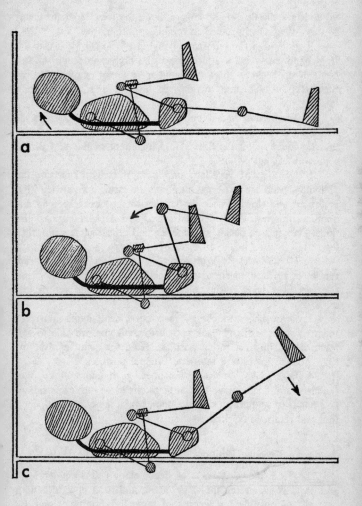

DIAGRAM 7

an arc until the tips of the fingers touch the toes. Hold for count of three then slowly return to original position.

19. Extend arms out from body at sides. Slowly raise the right hand, carry it in an arc above the body and touch the left hand. Keep heels on the floor. Hold for a count of three and return. Repeat, this time carrying the left hand across the body to the right.

20. With arms folded on chest, tighten abdominal muscles and raise head bringing chin toward chest. Now attempt to raise the shoulders up off the floor. Hold for count of five and slowly return to original position.

21. DIAGRAM 7: Clasp and hold the right knee on the abdomen, bend the left knee on abdomen, straighten left leg high in the air and slowly lower the left leg to the floor (keeping abdominal muscles tightened, head raised and back flat against the floor. Do not arch back). Change leg and repeat same with other leg.

22. DIAGRAM 8: With arms out to the side on floor, draw the knees upward to chest, then straighten the knees and swing the legs over head raising hips from the floor and return immediately.

23. Draw knees to chest, grasp knees with hands and pull them toward chest, roll back and forth until you are able to roll forward and up to a sitting position. Hold for count of five, release grip on knees and return to original position.

24. DIAGRAM 9: Raise the knees high and well up over the chest and head. Move legs in large circles as in bicycle riding. Use hands to support hips off the floor. Make ten circles with each foot and return to original position.

Assume a Kneeling Position, Then Sit Back on the Heels

25. Place hands at back of neck, elbows at shoulder level and back. Now, stretch the spine, chest, and head upward, sitting as "tall" as possible for a count of three; relax muscles and assume "slouched" position for count of three.

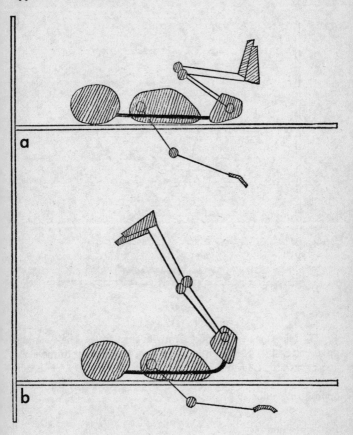

a

b

DIAGRAM 8

26. Place hands at back of neck, elbows forward in front of shoulders. Now, draw elbows, shoulders and head slowly backward as far as possible. Hold for count of three and resume original position.

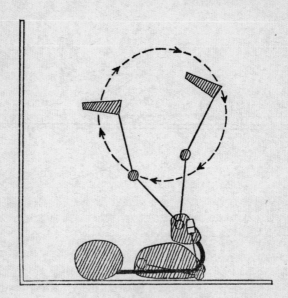

DIAGRAM 9

27. Place hands on hips, bend forward to an angle of approximately 45°. Now roll the body from the hips up to the right and backward, then to the left and finally forward; the head thus describing a circle in a clockwise direction. Repeat, going in the opposite direction.

Prone position

(Lie Face Downward on the Floor)

28. Bend the right leg at the knee as far as possible. Grasp with the right hand, hold for count of five and release. Repeat with the left leg.

29. DIAGRAM 10: Bend both legs at knees and grasp ankles with hands, raising chin off floor by arching back. Now rock back and forth five times, then relax.

30. Lie on abdomen, face down, arms at sides, shoulders high. Now, raise the head upward off the floor from the hips as high as possible. Hold for count of three and return to original position.

EXERCISES FOR THE NECK

Assume Correct Standing Position

1. Tip head back as far as possible. Keep lips together and chew hard, five times.

2. Hold head correctly and do not tilt chin, pull neck back in line with spine, keeping chin horizontal. Hold for count of five and return.

3. Bend head forward toward the chest as close as possible. Hold for the count of five and return.

4. Bend right ear toward right shoulder. Keep ear in line with shoulder. Hold for count of five and return to starting position. Repeat same toward left shoulder.

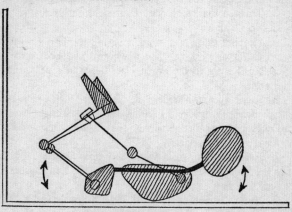

DIAGRAM 10

5. Turn face toward the right side as far as possible keeping the eyes level. Lead with your chin. Hold for the count of five and return to starting position. Repeat same toward left side.

6. Place hands on hips, keeping the rest of the trunk straight, bend the neck so as to place the chin as close to the chest as possible. Now, roll the head around to the right, to the back, to the left and finally to the forward position. Repeat in the opposite direction from left to right.

EXERCISES FOR THE SHOULDER

The following exercises are done standing erect and are started with the hands at the side.

1. Stand facing a mirror. Keeping the arms at the side, move the shoulders in a circular motion in the same direction.

2. DIAGRAM 11: Stand facing a mirror, somewhat less than arm's length from it. Place the tips of the fingers on the mirror and "walk up the mirror" with the hand. Watch in the mirror to make sure you are raising the arm at the shoulder—not elevating the shoulder or tilting the body. Hold for count of five at the highest point you can reach, then lower arm to side.

3. Turn so that your body is at right angles to the mirror. Repeat No. 2 above.

4. Keeping the elbow straight, swing the arm forward and upward as far as possible—then downward and backward as far as possible. Return to the original position and repeat using opposite arm.

5. Raise the arm sideward, shoulder high, palm down, make circles with the hand keeping the elbow straight; start with small circles and gradually increase the size of the circles. Do this first forward then backward.

6. Raise the arms sideward and upward, clapping hands above head, then lowering to the sides. Repeat, bringing the backs of hands together.

7. From the sitting position, fold arms across the chest, keeping elbows high. Now, unfold the arms, bringing the elbows

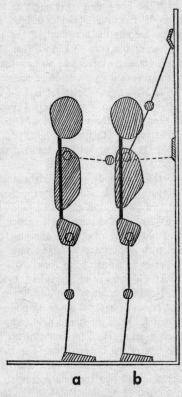

a   b

DIAGRAM 11

back, shoulders high, as far as possible. Hold for count of two and return.

8. Stand erect and place the hands behind the neck, palms forward. Now, quickly remove them from the neck; swing the arms down alongside the body and place the hands behind the lower back, palms facing backward; return quickly.

9. Stand with the body at a right angle to the wall. Grasp a bar or the edge of a door at shoulder height. Now, twist the body left and right, keeping the arm straight and in one place.

10. Grasp a bar or the edge of a door just above the head; slowly bend knees, gradually increasing pull on the arms.

11. With right arm resting on a table or counter and the body bent forward at the hips, right side to table, hold a weighted pail by the handle in the left hand. Swing the pail forward and backward ten times; then swing the pail from side to side ten times. Change hands, and repeat. (Increase weight, gradually, in pail.)

12. Repeat No. 11 above, but lean forward or sideways and swing pail in gradually increasing circles.

13. Stand so that the body is at a right angle to the wall, about an arm's length from it. Raise the arm closest to the wall to shoulder level and place palm of hand against the wall. Bend the elbow, lean to that side and attempt to touch the side of the head to the wall. Hold for count of three and push back to starting position. Repeat with opposite side facing wall.

14. Fold the arms in front of the chest. Now raise the arms as high as possible without raising shoulders, touching the forehead, if you can. Hold for count of two and return.

15. Clasp the hands in back of the neck, pulling elbows backward as far as possible. Hold the hands tight but bring the elbows forward and touch in front. Hold for count of two and return.

16. Place the tips of the fingers of one hand against the back of the head. Now, "crawl" down the neck and back as far as it will go. Hold for count of two and return slowly.

17. Place the back of one hand against the lower end of the spine, slide it upward along the backbone as far as it will go. Hold for count of two and return slowly.

18. Place both hands on the lower back. Pull the elbows forward as far as possible and then back as far as possible.

19. Flex the arms at the elbows so that forearms are parallel with the floor, palms turned in facing each other. Now, roll the shoulders in a circular shrugging motion, moving the arms back and forth (imitating the piston on a steam engine).

20. Lie face down on the side of your bed with one shoulder off the bed and that arm hanging down toward the floor. Swing the arm back and forth as far as possible.

21. Assume dorsal recumbent position. Now raise the arms in a circular motion and if possible, carry them all the way over the head and rest on the floor behind the head in a fully elevated position. Hold for count of three and return.

EXERCISES FOR THE ELBOW

1. Stand with hands at side, bend the elbows and touch the shoulders with the tips of the fingers. Hold for count of two and return to original position.

2. Repeat 1, holding dumbbell or other two-pound weight in hand.

3. Stand about two feet from a table. Lean forward and place palms of hands on table, about three feet apart. Continue to lean forward, bending the elbows and finally place chin on table. Hold for count of two and then push back to original position.

4. Sit in a chair and place the arm on a table in front of you, palm up. Now, roll the hand so that the palm is down. Hold for count of one and roll back.

5. Repeat No. 4 above but grasp a dumbbell or other two-pound weight in the hand. Hold this weight firmly while exercising.

6. DIAGRAM 12: Sit in a chair and place a bucket alongside the chair. Grasp the bucket and raise it, bending the elbow. When the arm is parallel to the floor, hold for count of two and return to original position. Increase the weight of the bucket by placing various objects in it.

7. Sit in an arm chair. Place the hands on the arms of the chair; push up against the arms of the chair straightening the elbows, lifting the hips from the seat. Hold for the count of one and return to the seat.

8. Generally, carry pocketbook or briefcase by the handle with the arms straight at the side.

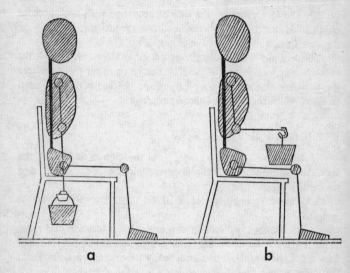

DIAGRAM 12

EXERCISES FOR THE WRIST

1. Sit in a chair or stool which has been placed in front of a sink or wash basin in the kitchen or bath room. Place a stopper in the drain and turn on the faucets so that the water will flow into the basin continuously and out the overflow. Adjust the temperature of the water so that it feels comfortably warm (about 100° to 105°). Now immerse the hands in the water above the wrists. Exercise the wrists through all motions possible. First, flex and extend them; then bend the hand in the direction of the thumb followed by bending in the direction of the little finger; finally, roll the hand at the wrist in an arc-like circular motion. Continue the exercising slowly and rhythmically 10-15 minutes, with a 15 second rest period each minute.

2. Close all fingers and thumb to a tight fist. Hold for count

of two and open to full extension, stretching the fingers as far apart as possible. Hold for count of two and relax.

3. Hold the arm extended in front of the body with fingers curled loosely, the palm facing the floor. Bend the hand at the wrist as far as possible and try to attain a right angle; bend so the palm of the hand faces the body. Hold for count of three. Now bend the hand in the opposite direction so that the palm faces forward, hold for count of three. Relax and return to the resting position with the hand and arm extended, the palm facing the floor.

4. Hold the arm extended in front of the body, with palm facing downward, index finger extended and other fingers curled loosely. Now, roll the hand on the wrist in a circular motion so that the index finger describes as large a circle as possible.

5. Grasp both handles of the doorknob. Twist with one hand, resisting with the other. Reverse.

6. Put the hand, palm downward, on the table. Place a folded newspaper or a light magazine across the back of the hand; flip it from the hand keeping the wrist on the table.

7. Rest the hand, palm upward on a table. Place a folded newspaper or a light magazine across ends of fingers. Now, keeping fingers rigid, flip it from the hand.

8. Face the wall. Place the palm of the hand against wall, shoulder high, with elbow bent and fingers pointing upward. Now slide arm downward against wall keeping fingers straight.

9. Hold a rod or pole firmly in both hands. Attempt to turn the pole in one direction with one hand and in the other direction with the other hand. Now reverse.

10. Using both hands, wring out assorted sizes of cloths.

11. Extend both arms upward, face palms together and interlock fingers. Now keeping fingers locked, bring the hands straight downward in front of the face and body as far as possible, keeping the palms facing the floor. If you can, carry the arms so that they now extend downward and palms face the floor. Hold for count of two and relax.

EXERCISES FOR THE FINGERS

1. Repeat exercise No. 1 under *Wrists*. Now exercise the fingers by flexing to a tight fist and extending forcefully to complete straightening of fingers.

2. Spread fingers far apart. Now make an "O" by touching tip of index finger to tip of thumb. Spread fingers far apart again. This time, make "O" by touching tip of middle finger to tip of thumb. Repeat, making "O" with tip of ring and little finger.

3. Make an "O" by touching tip of index finger to tip of thumb. Now, run index finger down thumb to its base and then up the thumb again to the tip. Repeat with each finger.

4. Reverse No. 3 above. Now, after making an "O" run the thumb down the index finger and back to the tip. Then repeat,

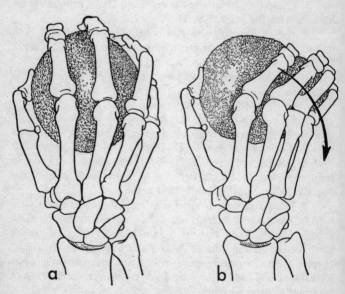

DIAGRAM 13

running the thumb down each of the other fingers and back to the tip.

5. Lay palm of hand flat on table. Now, raise and lower fingers one by one.

6. Crumple a full page of newspaper into a small ball with one hand.

7. Squeeze a small rubber ball or sponge. After each squeeze lay ball down and extend fingers as far as possible.

> CAUTION: Do not do this exercise if there is any deformity of wrist or fingers as it may increase the deformity (DIAGRAM 13).

8. Rest hand on table. Spread fingers wide and then bring them together.

9. Lay palm of hand flat on table. Now, flip paper balls with fingers, or flip a lightweight book or folded newspaper off extended fingers.

10. Extend arms in front of chest, palms together. Push against fingers of one hand with fingers of other. Now, reverse, pressing with fingers of opposite hand.

EXERCISES FOR THE KNEE JOINT

1. Perform exercise No. 15 listed under *Postural Exercises*.

2. From the dorsal recumbent position, bend the knees and bring the heels as close to the buttocks as possible. Support one thigh with the hands and extend the knee so that the leg is straight. Hold for count of three and return. Repeat with the opposite leg.

3. While sitting on the floor with legs straight in front, push knee down against floor tightening the thigh muscle and pulling the knee cap up toward the hips. Hold for count of seven and relax. Repeat with the opposite leg.

4. While in the dorsal recumbent position, place a rolled towel underneath the knees. Now contract the muscles of the legs so as to compress the towel against the floor as much as possible. Hold for the count of seven and relax.

5. Sit in a chair. Now, lift one thigh off the chair several inches. Extend the knee so as to straighten the leg as far as possible. Hold for a count of two, flex the knee to its original position and then let the thigh drop back onto the chair.

6. Sit on a table high enough so that the feet swing well off the floor. Hold a shopping bag on one of the feet with the loop or tie around the ankle, and place in it any object weighing about two pounds. Extend the knee so as to straighten the leg as far as possible. Hold for the count of two and return. Gradually increase the weight in the shopping bag.

7. Lie prone on the abdomen, face down and bend one knee. Make a complete turn of a sheet around the ankle, then grasp both ends of the sheet and attempt to bend the knee further by pulling very gently on the sheet.

8. Repeat No. 7 above, but instead of pulling on sheet to flex the knee, hold the sheet and attempt to straighten leg by extending the knee.

9. DIAGRAM 14: Stand at side of bed facing away from

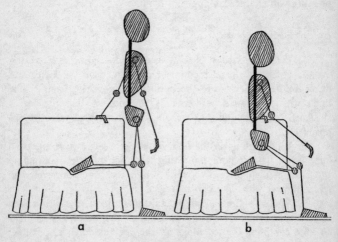

a   b

DIAGRAM 14

it. Hold on to the headboard. Bend one knee and place the lower leg on the bed. Now, slowly bend the body backwards and push downward against the foot as if you were going to sit on your foot. Hold for the count of two and return.

10. From standing position, gradually bend the knees, keeping the back straight, assume a squatting position. Hold for count of five and return.

EXERCISES FOR THE ANKLE JOINTS, FEET AND ARCHES

1. From the standing position, barefoot, raise the body as to stand on tiptoe. Hold for count of two and return to original position.

2. Walk slowly around the room on tiptoes.

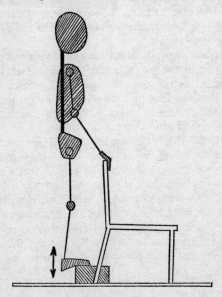

DIAGRAM 15

3. Walk around room on outside of feet, soles turned toward each other.

4. Place two chairs in front of you, back to back, and about two feet apart. Now stand between them with one foot about twelve inches in front of the other. While leaning forward and supporting some of the body weight on the chairs, raise heels and throw weight onto toes. Now, rock back onto heels. Continue rocking back and forth five times, gradually increasing weight on forward foot. Repeat, but reverse feet.

5. Stand facing a wall about an arm's length away. Lean forward and rest the hands on the wall. Keep the knees and hips straight and the heels flat on the floor. Bend elbows and try to touch chin to wall. Hold for count of three and return.

6. DIAGRAM 15: Stand on the edge of a low step or stool with the weight borne on the front part of the foot, heel off the edge. Try to let the heel drop below the level of the step, if possible. Hold onto some support and lower and raise the body weight up and down five times.

7. Sit in a chair. Raise the foot about six inches from the floor. Roll the foot at the ankle making a circle five times.

8. Sit in a chair and place six small pebbles or "playing jacks" on the floor. Pick up each pebble under the toes and carry it about a foot to the side and drop it. Return them to the original position with the opposite foot.

9. DIAGRAM 16: Sit in a chair and place a bandage or strap under the ball of the foot. Hold both ends with your hands. Pull up on the bandage, then resist and push foot down, curling toes under. Hold for count of three and relax.

10. Sit in a chair with knees bent, lower legs crossed and resting on the outer borders of feet. In this position, bend the toes under and curl tightly. Hold for count of three. Relax and then extend the toes as far as possible, bending in the opposite direction. Hold for count of three and assume resting position.

11. Sit in an arm chair; same position as No. 10 above. Rise from chair, supporting weight on the hands. Increase height of rise and reduce weight on hands. Rock from side to side on outer borders of feet.

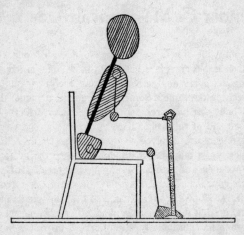

DIAGRAM 16

Appendix C: Mechanical Aids

Arthritis may, at times, impair the function of one or more joints. When this occurs, it is helpful to have some article to assist in carrying out every day activities. Many useful gadgets and devices have been developed. Some can be made at home; the more elaborate ones can be purchased from specialty dealers who are listed at the end of this appendix.

If the fingers are involved so that one has trouble closing his fist completely, he may find it difficult to grasp the average knife and fork—or pen and pencil. Wrapping the handles of such articles with gauze and tape may offer a simple and reasonable solution (DIAGRAM 17). One can also heat the handle of a knife or fork and drive it through a wax candle. Lengthening the handles of eating utensils (particularly the fork) will provide a better grip when cutting foods. It will also be helpful when there is trouble bringing food to the mouth because of restricted elbow motion. A "rocker knife" enables one to cut food with one hand when the second hand is not strong enough to hold a fork. When the elbow or shoulder motions are limited, a long handled comb, shoe horn and stocking aid may be invaluable when dressing, while long handled tongs may save the patient much bending and stooping.

Many arthritics develop weakness of the thigh muscles making it difficult to get up from a sitting position. And if the chair or toilet seat is rather low, this can become quite a problem. The solution here is to raise the seat so that the weakened quadriceps muscle will have less work (DIAGRAM 18).

If the joints of the lower extremities are involved, a cane or crutches may help to relieve the discomfort of walking. But proper selection and individual fitting are important.

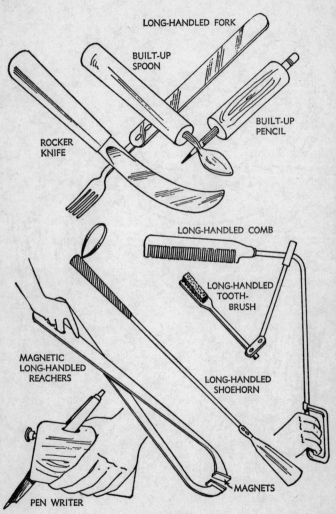

LONG-HANDLED FORK

BUILT-UP SPOON

BUILT-UP PENCIL

ROCKER KNIFE

LONG-HANDLED COMB

LONG-HANDLED TOOTH-BRUSH

MAGNETIC LONG-HANDLED REACHERS

LONG-HANDLED SHOEHORN

PEN WRITER

MAGNETS

DIAGRAM 17

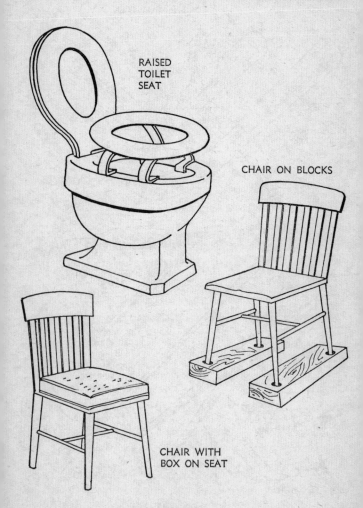

RAISED
TOILET
SEAT

CHAIR ON BLOCKS

CHAIR WITH
BOX ON SEAT

DIAGRAM 18

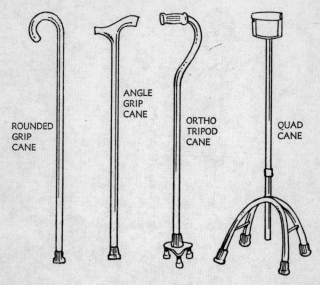

ROUNDED GRIP CANE

ANGLE GRIP CANE

ORTHO TRIPOD CANE

QUAD CANE

DIAGRAM 19

Canes: In choosing a cane, three factors are of importance—the handle or grip, the tip or foot, and the length. One should choose the grip which best fits his hand and which permits the firmest grasp to be maintained. The tip should be covered with a heavy gauge rubber pad to prevent slipping. It is usually single but may be "tripod" or "quadriped" to give greater stability. A cane is of the proper length when the tip touches the ground six inches in front of and to the side of the foot, and the forearm holding the cane makes a 30° angle at the elbow (DIAGRAM 20). The top of the cane will then usually be level with the upper level of the thigh bone.

Wooden canes when purchased are usually 36 inches long. They can be shortened as needed by removing the rubber tip, sawing to the desired length, and then replacing the tip. Adjustable aluminum canes are lighter but more expensive.

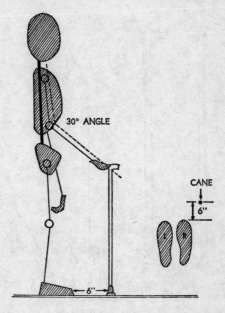

30° ANGLE

CANE

6"

6"

DIAGRAM 20

Crutches: Two quite distinct types of crutches are available (DIAGRAM 21). The underarm—or conventional; and the hand —or Lofstrand (so called after the American manufacturer who first popularized this type at the end of World War II). In general, women seem to prefer the former, men the latter. The Lofstrand crutch can only be used if the fingers and wrist are strong enough to support most of the body weight. A "platform" can be added to the conventional crutch or made into a separate crutch for those whose hands are too weak to support the weight in the usual manner. As with the selection of a cane, the proper crutch must be determined in consultation with your doctor, taking into consideration all factors of your arthritis.

Walking With a Cane or Crutch: If you watch a person walk,

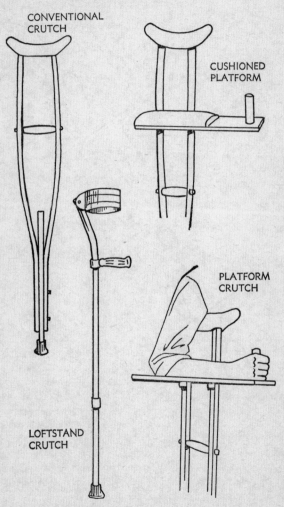

CONVENTIONAL CRUTCH

CUSHIONED PLATFORM

PLATFORM CRUTCH

LOFTSTAND CRUTCH

DIAGRAM 21

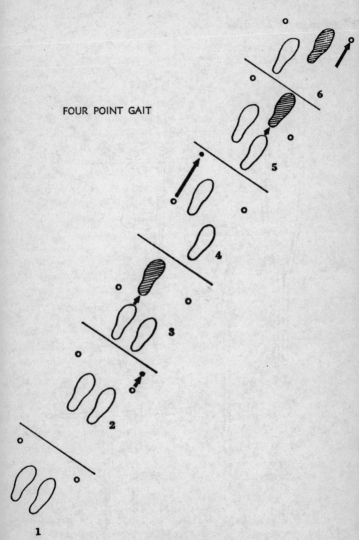

FOUR POINT GAIT

DIAGRAM 22

you will notice that his right arm swings forward as he advances his left foot, and vice versa. So it is natural when using a cane to hold it in the hand opposite the weak leg. In this way the weight of the body is shared between the cane and the arthritic leg as the "good" leg is lifted off the ground and advanced to take a step.

The same type of gait can be used with two canes or a pair of crutches. The left leg and the right arm holding a crutch are advanced. The weight is shifted to these, and the step is taken by throwing forward the right leg and left arm holding a crutch. Actually, this is a normal walking gait—assisted by canes or crutches. It is commonly referred to as a "two point" gait. When greater stability is needed a slower "four point" gait is used. This is illustrated in DIAGRAM 22 and is done as follows:

1. Stand with your weight distributed between your two feet and the two crutches (hence the four points).
2. Shift weight off the right crutch, lift it and carry it forward.
3. As a portion of the weight is shifted back onto the right crutch, the weight is taken off the left leg which is then moved forward to the desired step.
4. As the weight is again placed on the left foot, the weight is taken off the left crutch and it is moved forward.
5. As the weight goes back onto the left crutch, it is shifted off the right leg which in turn is advanced.
6. As the weight goes back on the right leg, the right crutch is again advanced, and the cycle repeated.

Although this may seem rather complicated, it really is not—a short practice session is usually all one needs to become quite adept.

Walkers: Walkers are now available which can be used with one or both hands. A "half-walker" may also come in quite handy under certain circumstances (DIAGRAM 23).

Back Braces: Some type of back support may be helpful in many conditions, ranging from simple sprains to collapsed vertebrae. The exact type of support to be prescribed is subject to

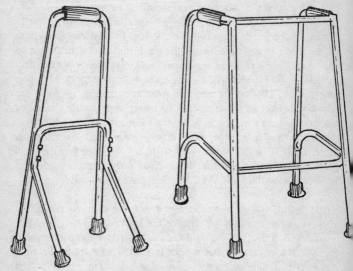

ALUMINUM WALKERS

DIAGRAM 23

so many individual factors that a full description would be impossible. The more common types of supports are shown in DIAGRAM 24.

SOURCES OF SELF-HELP AIDS

Surgical supply houses and many of the large drug stores in most cities will handle many of the aids described in this section. Persons who cannot find their needs met locally will be interested in the following:

1. Self-Help Devices: Rehabilitation Monograph XXI
An extremely comprehensive book of 193 pages showing, in pictures and text, all types of home and office helps for the handicapped. It is the result of years of study and work by Drs. Edward Lowman and Howard Rusk. Names of dealers from whom the

aids can be purchased are listed, but also included are tips on how to make many at home. The book can be purchased for $4.00 from—

> Publications Unit
> Institute of Rehabilitation Medicine
> New York University Medical Center
> 400 East 34th Street
> New York, New York 10016

2. The following firms either manufacture or distribute rehabilitation aids and will furnish prices on request. (Listed alphabetically):

A.   Cleo Living Aids
     3947 Mayfield Road
     Cleveland, Ohio 44121

B.   J. A. Preston Corporation
     71 Fifth Avenue
     New York, New York 10003

C.   Rehabilitation Products; Division of American Hospital
     Supply Corporation.
     Local offices are in most large cities and can be found
     in the telephone directory under either "Rehabilitation
     Products," or "American Hospital Supply Corporation."
     General office: 2020 Ridge Avenue
                          Evanston, Illinois

D.   Shalik's
     Box 612
     Tamiami Station
     Miami, Florida 33144

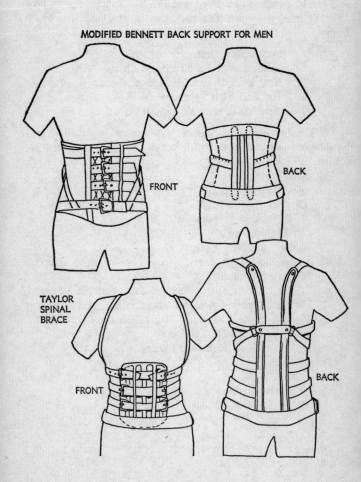

MODIFIED BENNETT BACK SUPPORT FOR MEN

FRONT

BACK

TAYLOR
SPINAL
BRACE

FRONT

BACK

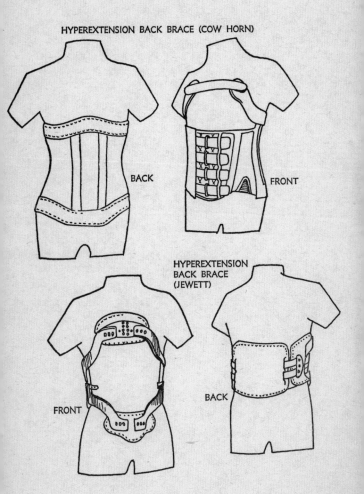

HYPEREXTENSION BACK BRACE (COW HORN)

BACK

FRONT

HYPEREXTENSION
BACK BRACE
(JEWETT)

FRONT

BACK

Index

Books on Health and Nutrition

VITAMIN E
Your Key to a Healthy Heart

Herbert Bailey

WHY IS VITAMIN E therapy for mankind's foremost killing disease still controversial in the United States? This is one of the questions asked and answered in this slashing, fully-documented book. It tells how the efficacy of vitamin E in the treatment of cardiovascular disease was discovered by Dr. Evan Shute of Canada, and of the remarkable cures effected by him and his brother, also a doctor . . . how the author himself suffered a severe heart attack and how in a short time he was restored to normal active life by massive doses of the vitamin . . . how a barrier against vitamin E has been erected in this country by the medical traditionalists of the American Medical Association at the same time that it is being widely used with spectacular results in such medically-advanced countries as England, Germany, France, Italy, and Russia . . . how continuing study indicates that vitamin E may be an effective preventive for diabetes, sterility, arthritis and a variety of other diseases. "Literally worth its weight in gold."
—**The Pittsburgh Courier**   **$1.65**

GET WELL NATURALLY

Linda Clark

LINDA CLARK believes that relieving human suffering and obtaining optimum health should be mankind's major goal. She insists that it does not matter whether a remedy is orthodox or unorthodox, currently praised or currently scorned in medical circles—as long as it works for you. Miss Clark, who is also the author of **Stay Young Longer,** makes a plea for the natural methods of treating disease—methods which do not rely on either drugs or surgery. Drawing not only from well-known sources but also from folklore and from the more revolutionary modern theories, she presents a wealth of information about diseases ranging from alcoholism to ulcers. Here are frank discussions of such controversial modes of treatment as herbal medicine, auto-therapy, homeopathy, and human electronics, plus some startling facts and theories about nutrition and about the natural ways of treating twenty-two of the most serious illnesses that plague modern man.   **$1.65**

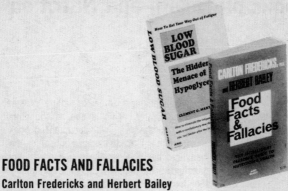

FOOD FACTS AND FALLACIES
Carlton Fredericks and Herbert Bailey

A noted nutritionist and veteran medical reporter present medical evidence based on modern research to prove that a good diet can lessen your effects of coming down with one of today's common health problems, such as heart disease, arthritis, mental illness, and many others. This book gives the unadulterated facts about fad diets, and it presents some startling information about proper diet and the prevention and treatment of alcoholism. To help you be sure that you are getting the balanced meals you need, the authors have included eleven rules for menu selection; tips on buying meats, cereals, and breads; lists of common sources of vitamins, carbohydrates, and fats; and an appendix of suggested menus. **$1.45**

LOW BLOOD SUGAR AND YOUR HEALTH
Eat Your Way Out of Fatigue
Clement G. Martin, M.D.

In this revolutionary new book, Dr. Martin tells exactly how to determine if hypoglycemia is the cause of fatigue problems, and if so, he outlines a diet that can make anyone feel better after the first week. It's not a starvation diet, not a fad diet. But it is unusual. The Doctor instructs the reader to eat eight times a day rather than three. And for those who don't suffer from hypoglycemia, it is still probable that the cause of the fatigue or mental distress is nutrition. These people will find Dr. Martin's delicious, eight-times-a-day diet pouring new energy into their bodies.

This is not a book of "miracle cures." It is a book about common sense attitudes toward nutrition and exercise—proof positive that a sensible, well-balanced diet is the **real** key to good health. **$1.65**

ORGANIC GARDENING AND FARMING

Joseph A. Cocannouer

A blueprint for soil management designed to enable you to grow better-testing, healthful, fruits, vegetables and other food crops. Here is complete information on **organic** gardening and farming—gardening without poisonous pesticides—where to start, what to do and how to follow through whether in a window box, backyard or on acres of soil. Everything you need to know to make friends with the earth the natural way is included—organic soil conditioners, composts and mulches, pest control without poison, tips on planting and landscaping.
Clothbound: $4.50
Paperbound: $1.45

NATURE'S MIRACLE MEDICINE CHEST

C. Edward Burtis

How to achieve abundant good health through everyday wonder foods—pure natural foods, our gifts from the land and sea. Mr. Burtis covers many of the wonder foods found in nature's miracle medicine chest and explains how to use them for better health—the fantastic papaya melon, digestive disorders and the lime, slipped discs and vitamin C, cabbage juice and ulcers, yogurt and digestive health, calcium and the heart, bone meal and loose teeth, garlic and diarrhea, the bactericidal qualities of honey, the remarkable powers of royal jelly, kelp for the common cold, cod liver oil and arthritis, vitamin E and the heart, brewer's yeast as a protective agent, sesame seeds as a tranquilizer.
Clothbound, $5.95

COMMON AND UNCOMMON USES OF HERBS FOR HEALTHFUL LIVING

Richard Lucas

A fascinating account of the herbal remedies used through the ages. Plant medicine has been used for thousands of years and modern science is now re-evaluating many old-time herbal medicines. Described here are the herbal folk remedies that have been used for centuries by the American Indians, the gypsies, the ancient herbalists, the countryfolk, and the old-time country doctor. The background, history and uses of such healing herbs as dandelion, elder, nettle, sage, kelp, onion, parsley, sassafras, rosemary, camomile, corn silk, celery as cures for rash, hives, urinary disorders, ulcers, gout, and nervous disorders are described. **$1.65**

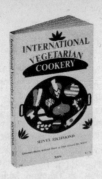 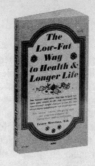 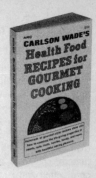

THE LOW-FAT WAY TO HEALTH AND LONGER LIFE

Lester Morrison, M.D.

The famous best-seller that has helped millions gain robust health and increased life span through simple changes in diet, the use of nutritional supplements and weight control. With menus, recipes, life-giving diets, and programs endorsed by distinguished medical authorities. **$1.65**

CARLSON WADE'S HEALTH FOOD RECIPES FOR GOURMET COOKING Carlson Wade

Hundreds of recipes for preparing natural health foods—gourmet style—for healthful eating pleasure. The secret of youthful energy and vitality is in the magical powers of vitamins, minerals, enzymes, protein, and other life-giving elements found in **natural foods.** In this new book, noted nutrition expert Carlson Wade shows you how you can make delicious meals prepared with pure, natural foods; seeds, nuts, berries, whole grains, honey, fruits, fish and more. **$1.65**

INTERNATIONAL VEGETARIAN COOKERY

Sonya Richmond

This book proves that vegetarian cookery, far from being dull and difficult to prepare, can open up completely new and delightful vistas of haute cuisine. Miss Richmond, who has traveled throughout the world, has arranged the book alphabetically according to countries, starting with Austria and going through to the United States. She gives recipes for each country's most characteristic vegetarian dishes and lists that country's outstanding cheeses.

Clothbound: $3.75
Paperbound: $1.75

HOW TO BE HEALTHY WITH NATURAL FOODS

Edward G. Marsh

Do you feel sluggish, tired, old beyond your years? Do you get frequent colds, lack pep and energy, feel overweight and stuffed? Chances are that you are not eating the right foods. The average American's diet today consists of innutritious processed foods, fats and starches, insufficient vitamins and minerals—a diet that contains little or nothing of value and, usually, much that is downright harmful. **HOW TO BE HEALTHY WITH NATURAL FOODS** shows that it is possible to maintain optimum health and eliminate colds and other chronic ailments by using only wholesome, natural foods and by eliminating from your diet foods that are harmful or that contain nothing of value to your body. In this concise, practical book on nutrition, the author presents simple, tried and tested rules for the selection of healthful and tasty foods, including suggestions for specific diets to build and maintain vitality, protect against senility, and promote vigorous health and long life. **$1.45**

THE SOYBEAN COOKBOOK

Mildred Lager & Dorothea Van Gundy Jones

Soybeans . . . almost as old as civilization . . . are today the newest and most exciting phenomenon in the nutrition field. This book fills the urgent need for a comprehensive cookbook dealing with this nutritious and versatile food. Included here are over 350 recipes for delicious ways to use soybeans in dishes ranging from salads to souffles to desserts. Each recipe has many zestful variations, and the book offers suggestions for using the beans in all their many forms, including soy flour, dried soybeans, cooked green soybeans, soy oil, and soy sprouts. Also included is a discussion of the soybean's nutritional value and a brief history of its uses. **Clothbound: $4.50**
Paperbound: $1.45

HEALTH FOODS AND HERBS

Kathleen Hunter

The advantages of eating only natural foods are discussed in this comprehensive guide to healthful living. Included are many easy-to-prepare recipes made with mushrooms, yogurt, cheese, fresh vegetables, seaweed, nuts, honey, and other untreated foods plus extensive information on using herbs—both for medicinal and culinary purposes. Miss Hunter also discusses the important vitamin groups, chemical fertilizers, and the safest types of cooking utensils. **Clothbound: $4.50**
Paperbound: 95c

HEALTH, FITNESS, and MEDICINE BOOKS

All books are available at your bookseller or directly from ARCO PUBLISHING COMPANY INC., 219 Park Avenue South, New York, N.Y. 10003. Send price of books plus 25¢ for postage and handling. No C.O.D.